Practical Handbook of OCT Angiography

Editors

Bruno Lumbroso MD
Director, Centro Italiano Macula
Former Director
Rome Eye Hospital
Rome, Italy

David Huang MD PhD
Peterson Professor
Department of Ophthalmology
Professor, Biomedical Engineering
Casey Eye Institute
Oregon Health and Science University
Portland, USA

Eric Souied MD PhD
Professor and Head
Department of Ophthalmology
Centre Hospitalier Intercommunal de Creteil
Université Paris Est Créteil
Créteil, France

Marco Rispoli MD
Staff Ophthalmologist
Department of Ophthalmology
Ospedale Nuova Regina Margherita
Centro Italiano Macula
Rome, Italy

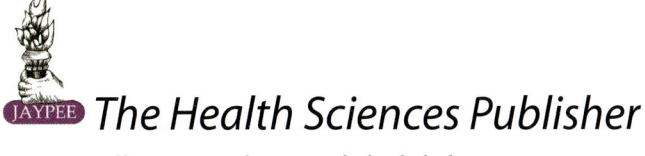

JAYPEE *The Health Sciences Publisher*

New Delhi | London | Philadelphia | Panama

Jaypee Brothers Medical Publishers (P) Ltd.

Headquarters
Jaypee Brothers Medical Publishers (P) Ltd.
4838/24, Ansari Road, Daryaganj
New Delhi 110 002, India
Phone: +91-11-43574357
Fax: +91-11-43574314
E-mail: jaypee@jaypeebrothers.com

Overseas Offices

J.P. Medical Ltd.	Jaypee-Highlights Medical Publishers Inc.	JP Medical Inc.
83, Victoria Street, London	City of Knowledge, Bld. 235, 2nd Floor, Clayton	325, Chestnut Street
SW1H 0HW (UK)	Panama City, Panama	Suite 412
Phone: +44-20 3170 8910	Phone: +1 507-301-0496	Philadelphia, PA 19106, USA
Fax: +44(0) 20 3008 6180	Fax: +1 507-301-0499	Phone: +1 267-519-9789
E-mail: info@jpmedpub.com	E-mail: cservice@jphmedical.com	E-mail: support@jpmedus.com

Jaypee Brothers Medical Publishers (P) Ltd.
17/1-B, Babar Road, Block-B, Shaymali
Mohammadpur, Dhaka-1207
Bangladesh
Mobile: +08801912003485
E-mail: jaypeedhaka@gmail.com

Jaypee Brothers Medical Publishers (P) Ltd.
Bhotahity, Kathmandu, Nepal
Phone: +977-9741283608
E-mail: kathmandu@jaypeebrothers.com

Website: www.jaypeebrothers.com
Website: www.jaypeedigital.com

© 2016, Jaypee Brothers Medical Publishers

The views and opinions expressed in this book are solely those of the original contributor(s)/author(s) and do not necessarily represent those of editor(s) of the book.

All rights reserved. No part of this publication may be reproduced, stored or transmitted in any form or by any means, electronic, mechanical, photocopying, recording or otherwise, without the prior permission in writing of the publishers.

All brand names and product names used in this book are trade names, service marks, trademarks or registered trademarks of their respective owners. The publisher is not associated with any product or vendor mentioned in this book.

Medical knowledge and practice change constantly. This book is designed to provide accurate, authoritative information about the subject matter in question. However, readers are advised to check the most current information available on procedures included and check information from the manufacturer of each product to be administered, to verify the recommended dose, formula, method and duration of administration, adverse effects and contraindications. It is the responsibility of the practitioner to take all appropriate safety precautions. Neither the publisher nor the author(s)/editor(s) assume any liability for any injury and/or damage to persons or property arising from or related to use of material in this book.

This book is sold on the understanding that the publisher is not engaged in providing professional medical services. If such advice or services are required, the services of a competent medical professional should be sought.

Every effort has been made where necessary to contact holders of copyright to obtain permission to reproduce copyright material. If any has been inadvertently overlooked, the publisher will be pleased to make the necessary arrangements at the first opportunity.

Inquiries for bulk sales may be solicited at: jaypee@jaypeebrothers.com

Practical Handbook of OCT Angiography

First Edition: **2016**
ISBN: 978-93-85999-97-0
Printed at Replika Press Pvt. Ltd.

Contributors

Ala El Ameen MD
Department of Ophthalmology
Centre Hospitalier Intercommunal de Creteil
Université Paris Est Créteil
Creteil, France

Luca Di Antonio MD PhD
Retina Fellow
Department of Ophthalmology
University G d'Annunzio of Chieti-Pescara, Italy

Vittorio Capuano MD
Department of Ophthalmology
Centre Hospitalier Intercommunal de Creteil
Université Paris Est Créteil
Creteil, France

Salomon Yves Cohen MD
Department of Ophthalmology
Centre Hospitalier Intercommunal de Creteil
Université Paris Est Créteil
Creteil, France

Eliana Costanzo MD
Department of Ophthalmology
Centre Hospitalier Intercommunal
de Creteil
Université Paris Est Créteil
Creteil, France

Adil El Maftouhi OD
Centre Rabelais, Lyon
XV XX Hospital
Service du Pr C. Baudouin
Paris, France

Simon S Gao PhD
Postdoctoral Fellow
Casey Eye Institute
Oregon Health and Science University
Portland, USA

David Huang MD PhD
Peterson Professor
Department of Ophthalmology
Professor, Biomedical Engineering
Casey Eye Institute
Oregon Health and Science University
Portland, USA

Yali Jia PhD
Research Assistant Professor
Casey Eye Institute
Oregon Health and Science University
Portland, USA

Jean François Le Rouic MD
Department of Vitreo Retinal Surgery
Clinique Sourdille, Nantes, France

Bruno Lumbroso MD
Director, Centro Italiano Macula
Former Director
Rome Eye Hospital, Rome, Italy

Leonardo Mastropasqua MD PhD
Professor and Head
Department of Ophthalmology
University G d'Annunzio of Chieti-Pescara
Center of Excellence
National High-tech Center (CNAT) and Italian
School of Robotic Surgery in Ophthalmology
Italy

Alexandra Miere MD
Department of Ophthalmology
Centre Hospitalier Intercommunal de Creteil
Université Paris Est Creteil
Créteil, France

Pascal Peronnet MD
Clinique Sourdille
Nantes, France

Michel Puech MD FRSC
Explore Vision
VuExplorer Institute
Paris, France

Maddalena Quaranta-El Maftouhi MD
Centre Ophthalmologique Rabelais
Lyon, France

Giuseppe Querques MD PhD
Head
Medical Retina and Imaging Unit
Department of Ophthalmology
University Vita Salute
San Raffaele Scientific Institute
Milan, Italy

Marco Rispoli MD
Staff Ophthalmologist
Department of Ophthalmology
Ospedale Nuova Regina Margherita
Centro Italiano Macula
Rome, Italy

Maria Cristina Savastano MD PhD
Centro Italiano Macula
Rome, Italy

Oudy Semoun MD
Department of Ophthalmology
Centre Hospitalier Intercommunal de Creteil
Université Paris Est Créteil
Creteil, France

Eric Souied MD PhD
Professor and Head
Department of Ophthalmology
Centre Hospitalier Intercommunal de Creteil
Université Paris Est Créteil
Créteil, France

Preface

Twenty years after the unanimous acceptance of structural optical coherence tomography (OCT), the OCT devices find their place in every ophthalmological examination room alongside the slit lamp.

The functional OCT angiography has been clinically available only for the last two years, but its use is spreading explosively all over the world, and beginning to replace, in most conditions, the invasive fluorescein angiography. This new non-invasive technology is faster, easier, less expensive and can be repeated frequently without problems for the patient.

The only problem for the beginner is that the imaging is different from fluorescein imaging. It is necessary to learn a different interpretation modality. Acquisition of images is an important step, but imaging interpretation is the subsequent most important step.

The incessant succession of technological progresses and improvements in the field of imaging *oblige the ophthalmologist and the imaging technician to a continuous updating effort, without which they will lag behind our specialty evolution.* This book is conceived to help them.

I had the honor to write this book with:
- David Huang, one of the co-inventors of OCT, as well as co-inventor, with Yali Jia, of split-spectrum amplitude-decorrelation angiography (SSADA) technology of OCT angiography;
- Eric Souied, eminent clinician, geneticist and imaging specialist; and
- Marco Rispoli, a leading expert and pioneer in OCT angiography and ocular imaging.

Bruno Lumbroso

Acknowledgments

Our thanks to Jay Wei, CEO of Optovue, who encouraged us to write a practical guide to OCT angiography, for many years of friendly collaboration.

Our gratitude to Judy Bartlett-Roberto for the help in revising the text.

Contents

1. **Principles of Optical Coherence Tomography Angiography** 1
   David Huang, Yali Jia, Simon S Gao
   - Optical Coherence Tomography Angiography 1

2. **Interpretation of Optical Coherence Tomography Angiography** 6
   David Huang, Yali Jia, Simon S Gao
   - Anatomic Reference Planes and Angiographic Slabs 6
   - AngioVue Default Segmentation and Display 8

3A. **Quantification of Vascular Layers with Optical Coherence Tomography Angiography** 16
   Marco Rispoli
   - Flow Area 16
   - Nonflow Area (Vascular Dropout Area) 16
   - Flow Density Map 16

3B. **Practical Problems and Artifacts in Optical Coherence Tomography Angiography** 22
   Marco Rispoli, Bruno Lumbroso

4. **Optical Coherence Tomography Angiography of Normal Retina and its Vascular Structure** 24
   Maria Cristina Savastano, Marco Rispoli, Bruno Lumbroso
   - Retinal Vascular Networks 24

5. **Diabetic Retinopathy and Optical Coherence Tomography Angiography** 28
   Maria Cristina Savastano, Marco Rispoli, Bruno Lumbroso
   - Objective Quantitative Analysis 32

6. **Vascular Occlusions** 33
   Marco Rispoli, Bruno Lumbroso, Maria Cristina Savastano, Jean Francois Le Rouic, Pascal Peronnet

   Branch or Central Vein Occlusions 33
   Marco Rispoli, Bruno Lumbroso, Maria Cristina Savastano
   - Central Retinal Vein Occlusion and Venous Branch Occlusion 33
   - Optical Coherence Tomography Angiography 34

   Retinal Artery Occlusion 40
   Jean Francois Le Rouic, Pascal Peronnet
   - Retinal Artery Occlusion: Acute Stage 40
   - Retinal Artery Occlusion: Late Phase 41
   - Treatment 42

7. **Type 1, Type 2 and Type 4 (Mixed) Choroidal Neovascularization** 44
   Bruno Lumbroso, Marco Rispoli
   - Assessing New Vessels 45
   - Type 1 New Vessels 45

- Type 2 New Vessels 47
- Type 3 New Vessels 50
- Type 4 New Vessels (Mixed Type) 50
- Neovascular Membranes in Myopia 52

8. **Type 3 Neovascularization Features on Optical Coherence Tomography Angiography** — 56
   Alexandra Miere, Giuseppe Querques, Ala El Ameen, Vittorio Capuano, Oudy Semoun, Eric Souied

9. **Choroidal Neovascularization in Diseases other than Age-related Macular Degeneration** — 61
   Adil El Maftouhi, Maddalena Quaranta-El Maftouhi

   Degenerative Myopia, CSC, Multiple Choroiditis — 61
   Adil El Maftouhi, Maddalena Quaranta-El Maftouhi
   - Degenerative Myopia 61
   - Choroidal New Vessel Complications in Angioid Streaks 61
   - Chronic Central Serous Chorioretinopathy 61
   - Choroidal New Vessel Complications in Multifocal Choroiditis 62

   Polypoidal Choroidal Vasculopathy — 77
   Maddalena Quaranta-El Maftouhi, Adil El Maftouhi

10. **Other Types of Choroidal Neovascularization not Linked to Age-related Macular Degeneration** — 87
    Leonardo Mastropasqua, Luca Di Antonio

11. **Subretinal Fibrosis Features in Optical Coherence Tomography Angiography** — 93
    Eric Souied, Alexandra Miere, Oudy Semoun, Eliana Costanzo, Salomon Yves Cohen

12. **Evolution in Time of Flows after Treatment** — 98
    Bruno Lumbroso, Marco Rispoli
    - Early Changes after Treatment 98

13. **Optic Nerve and Glaucoma** — 103
    Michel Puech
    - Optical Coherence Tomography Angiography around the Optic Disc 103
    - Vascularization Inside the Optic Disc 104

14. **Comparing Fluorescein Angiography with Optical Coherence Tomography Angiography** — 107
    Bruno Lumbroso, Marco Rispoli
    - Fluorescein Angiography 107

Index — 115

Introduction

Practical Handbook of OCT Angiography deals with optical coherence tomography (OCT) angiography, a revolutionary development in ocular imaging. In it, we offer a step-by-step guide for interpreting the new images and data acquired by OCT angiography. It uses a logical method for interpreting ophthalmic images and will inform clinicians and technicians on the recent advances in OCT angiography imaging.

The new, non-invasive, dyeless OCT angiography is taking an important place as a diagnostic tool in everyday ophthalmology, as complement of, and, in part, replacing fluorescein angiography. OCT angiography technology allows for studying inner and outer retina disorders, both qualitatively and quantitatively, and classifying choroidal neovascularization (CNV) in a non-invasive manner, highlighting morphology, flow and depth. It gives new technical and clinical information in the study of glaucoma.

This book subdivides each image into its elementary identifiable features and then combines elementary components to synthesize the data, allowing diagnosis and treatment decision.

All imaging in this book has been obtained from Optovue's Avanti Widefield OCT hardware platform and AngioVue OCT angiography software. The Avanti is a spectral-domain OCT with the high speed necessary for angiography. The AngioVue software incorporates the highly efficient split-spectrum amplitude-decorrelation angiography (SSADA) algorithm that allows for high-quality wide-area angiograms to be acquired in less than 3 seconds. A very useful new software named AngioAnalytics gives numerical measurements on vessel area and vessel density map that is especially helpful on follow-up examinations, enabling quantitative comparison with the baseline values.

We trust this book will help ophthalmologists, residents, ophthalmic technicians and optometrists to understand and appreciate the new possibilities offered by OCT angiography imaging.

Bruno Lumbroso
David Huang
Eric Souied
Marco Rispoli

1

Principles of Optical Coherence Tomography Angiography

David Huang, Yali Jia, Simon S Gao

Optical coherence tomography (OCT) has become part of the standard of care in ophthalmology. It provides cross-sectional and three-dimensional (3D) imaging of the anterior segment, retina, and optic nerve head with micrometer-scale depth resolution. Structural OCT enhances the clinician's ability to detect and monitor fluid exudation associated with vascular diseases. It, however, is unable to directly detect capillary dropout or pathologic vessel growth (neovascularization) that constitute the major vascular change associated with two leading causes of blindness, age-related macular degeneration and diabetic retinopathy. These features, among other vascular abnormalities, are assessed clinically using fluorescein or indocyanine green (ICG) angiography. To overcome conventional structural OCT's inability to provide direct blood flow information, several OCT angiography methods have been developed.

OPTICAL COHERENCE TOMOGRAPHY ANGIOGRAPHY

Initially, Doppler OCT angiography methods were investigated for the visualization and measurement of blood flow.[1-6] Because Doppler OCT is sensitive only to motion parallel to the OCT probe beam, it is limited in its ability to image retinal and choroidal circulation, which are predominantly perpendicular to the OCT beam. An alternative approach has been speckle-based OCT angiography. It has advantages over Doppler-based techniques because it uses the variation of the speckle pattern in time to detect both transverse and axial flow with similar sensitivities. Amplitude-based,[7-9] phase-based,[10] or combined amplitude+phase[11] variance methods have been described.

Split-spectrum Amplitude-decorrelation Angiography

We developed an amplitude-based method called split-spectrum amplitude-decorrelation angiography (SSADA). The SSADA algorithm detects motion in blood vessel lumen by measuring the variation in reflected OCT signal amplitude between consecutive cross-sectional scans. Decorrelation is a mathematical function that quantifies variation without being affected by the average signal strength, as long as the signal is strong enough to predominate over optical and electronic noise. This novelty of SSADA lies in how the OCT signal is processed to enhance flow detection and reject axial bulk motion noise. Specifically, the algorithm splits the OCT image into different spectral bands, thus increasing the number of usable image frames. Each new frame has a lower axial resolution that is less susceptible to axial eye motion caused by retrobulbar pulsation. This lower resolution also translates to a wider coherence gate over which reflected signal from a moving particle such as a blood cell can interfere with adjacent structures, thereby increasing speckle contrast. In addition, each spectral band contains a different speckle pattern and independent information on flow. When amplitude decorrelation images from multiple spectral bands are combined, the flow signal is increased. Compared to the full-spectrum amplitude method, SSADA using four-fold spectral splits improved the signal-to-noise ratio (SNR) by a factor of two, which is equivalent to reducing the scan time by a factor of four.[12] More recent SSADA implementations use even more than a four-fold split to further enhance the SNR of flow detection. As shown by an example from *en face* angiograms of the macular retinal circulation collected using a commercial 70 kHz 840-nm spectral OCT **(Figs 1.1A to H)**, SSADA provides a clean and continuous microvascular network and less noise just inside the foveal avascular zone (FAZ).

Since OCT angiography generates 3D data, segmentation and *en face* presentation of the flow information can aid in reducing data complexity and serve to reproduce the more traditional view of dye-based angiography. As seen in **Figure 1.1**, the retinal angiogram **(Figs 1.1B to D)** represents the decorrelation or flow information between the internal limiting membrane and the outer plexiform layer. Segmentation performed on the cross-sectional, structural OCT images **(Fig. 1.1E)** can directly be applied to the OCT angiography images **(Figs 1.1F and G)**. The *en face* angiograms were generated by projecting the maximum decorrelation or flow value for each transverse position within the segmented depth range, representing the fastest flowing vessel lumen in the segmented tissue layers. In healthy eyes, the retinal angiogram shows a vascular network around the FAZ. The layers of the retina and choroid can

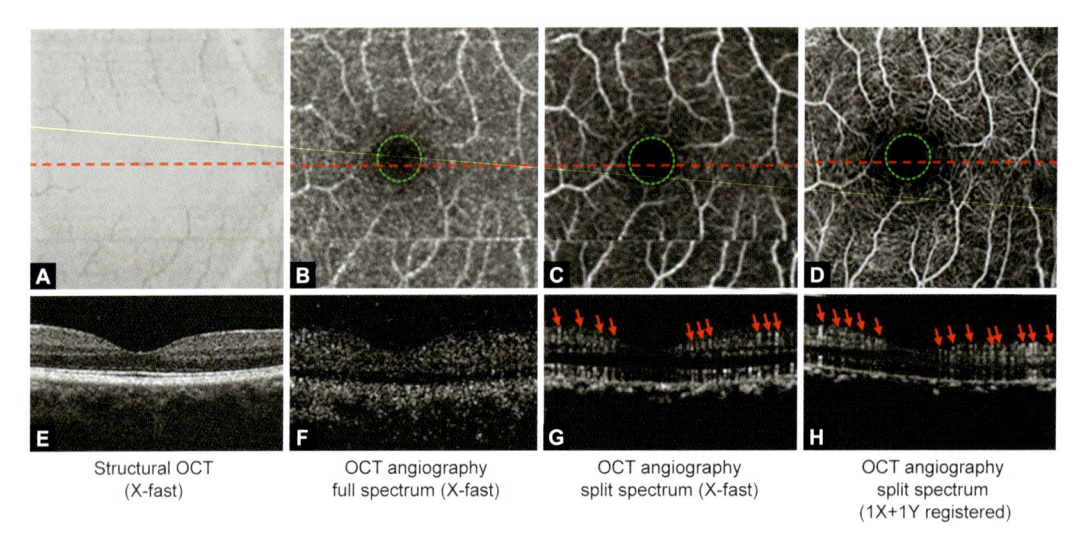

Figures 1.1A to H Comparison of structural optical coherence tomography (OCT) (A, E) and amplitude-decorrelation angiograms of the macula (3 × 3 mm area) using full spectrum (B, F), split-spectrum (C, G), and split-spectrum averaged angiograms from one X-fast and one F-fast scans after 3D registration (D, H). *En face* maximum decorrelation projections of retinal circulation showed less noise inside the foveal avascular zone (FAZ, within green dotted circles) and more continuous perifoveal vascular networks using the split-spectrum amplitude-decorrelation angiography (SSADA) algorithm (C) compared to standard full-spectrum algorithm (B). The cross-sectional angiograms (scanned across the red dashed line in B and C) showed more clearly delineated retinal vessels (red arrows in G) and less noise using the SSADA algorithm (G) compared to the standard (F). There are saccadic motion artifacts that appear as artifactual horizontal lines in (B, C). This and other motion artifacts are removed using the 3D registration algorithm that registers a horizontal-priority (X-fast) and a vertical-priority (Y-fast) raster scans to remove motion error. The algorithm then merges the X-fast and Y-fast scans to produce a merged 3D OCT angiogram that shows a continuous artifact-free microvascular network in (D). The registration and averaging of two orthogonal scans also removed motion blur and further improved SNR, allowing the visualization of a greater number of distinct small retinal vessels (microvascular network in D, red arrows in H)
Abbreviation: OCT, optical coherence tomography

be more finely separated to provide additional information to define diagnostic parameters of vascular defects. This will be discussed in Chapter 2.

Relationship Between Decorrelation and Velocity

To determine how the decorrelation or flow signal produced by the SSADA algorithm relates to flow velocity, phantom experiments were performed.[13] The study showed that SSADA is sensitive to both axial and transverse flow, with a slightly higher sensitivity for the axial component. For clinical retinal imaging, where the OCT beam is approximately perpendicular to the vasculature, the SSADA signal can be considered to be independent of the small variation in beam incidence angle for all practical purposes. In addition, it was found that decorrelation was linearly related to velocity over a limited range. A higher decorrelation value thus, implies higher velocity flow. This range is dependent on the time scale of the SSADA measurement. With a 70 kHz spectral OCT system and 200+ A-scans per cross-sectional B-scan, SSADA should be sensitive to even the slowest flow at the capillary level, where flow speeds have been estimated at between 0.4 and 3 mm/s.[14,15] In larger vessels with higher velocities, the SSADA signal reaches a maximum value (saturates).

Comparison to Fluorescein and Indocyanine Green Angiography

Compared to fluorescein or ICG angiography, the gold standards of retinal vascular imaging, OCT angiography has a number of advantages and differences. SSADA can be acquired in a few seconds and does not require intravenous injection, whereas fluorescein or ICG angiography requires multiple image frames taken over several minutes and can cause nausea, vomiting, and, albeit rarely, anaphylaxis.[16] The fast and noninvasive nature of OCT angiography also means that follow-ups scans can be conducted more frequently.

Dye leakage in fluorescein angiography is the hallmark of important vascular abnormalities such as neovascularization and microaneurysms. OCT angiography does not employ a dye and cannot evaluate leakage. OCT angiography detects vascular abnormalities by other methods based on depth and vascular pattern. Choroidal neovascularization is characterized by distinct vascular patterns present above the retinal pigment epithelium (Type II) or between the Bruch's membrane and the retinal pigment epithelium (Type I). Because dye leakage and staining do not occur in OCT angiography, the boundaries, and therefore areas, of capillary dropout and neovascularization can be more precisely measured. The visualization of intraretinal and subretinal fluid accumulation on structural OCT may provide information analogous to fluid leakage. Thus, although the lack of dye leakage is a limitation of OCT angiography, other ways of detecting vascular abnormality more than make up for this deficit. Furthermore, conventional angiography is two-dimensional, which makes it difficult to distinguish vascular abnormalities within different layers. The 3D nature of OCT angiography allows for separate evaluation of abnormalities in the retinal and choroidal circulations.

Limitations of Optical Coherence Tomography Angiography

The OCT angiography has several limitations. First, shadowgraphic flow projection artifact makes the interpretation of *en face* angiograms of deeper vascular beds more difficult. These artifacts are a result of fluctuating shadows cast by flowing blood in a superficial vascular layer that cause variation of the OCT signal in deeper, highly reflective layers. The flow projection artifact from the retinal circulation can be seen clearly on the bright retinal pigment epithelium (RPE). This artifact can be removed by software processing. The projection from the retinal circulation is relatively sparse and can be removed from deeper layers fairly effectively. However, the choriocapillaris is nearly confluent, and its projection and shadow effects are difficult to remove from deeper choroidal layers. A second limitation is the fading of OCT and flow signal in large vessels due to the interferometric fringe washout effect associated with very fast blood flow, especially the axial flow component.[17] This means that central retinal vessels in the disc and large vessels in the deep choroid cannot be

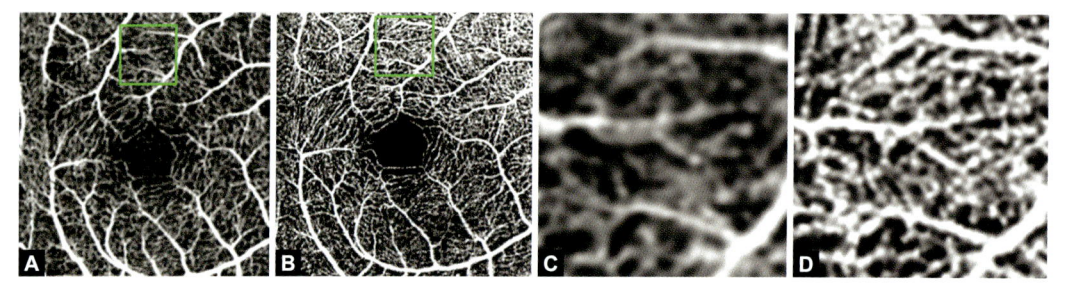

Figures 1.2A to D Comparison of 3 × 3 mm macular angiograms from a 100 kHz swept-source OCT system (A) and 70 kHz spectral OCT system (B) as compared to the swept-source OCT system (C) Zoomed-in views shows improve capillary detail from the spectral OCT system (D)

visualized using SSADA. Third, the scan area of OCT angiography is relatively small (3 × 3 to 6 × 6 mm). Larger-area angiograms of high quality can be achieved, but require higher speed OCT systems that are not yet commercially available.[18] Lastly, because OCT angiography best resolves pathology when viewed as *en face* angiograms of anatomic layers, practical clinical applications require accurate segmentation software. Post-processing software is also needed to reduce motion and projection artifacts. The need for these sophisticated algorithms means OCT angiography still has much room to improve in the foreseeable future.

Comparing Swept-source and Spectral Optical Coherence Tomography

The SSADA algorithm was initially implemented on a custom-built 100 kHz 1050 nm wavelength swept-source OCT system. To generate high quality angiograms **(Fig. 1.2A)**, 8 consecutive cross-sectional scan at each position were necessary. A scan pattern of 200 cross-sectional scan positions each with 200 axial scans was used. The overall angiographic scan pattern had 200 × 200 transverse points. The total of 200 × 200 × 8 axial scans were acquired in 3.5 seconds.

The commercial implementation of SSADA uses a 70 kHz 840 nm wavelength spectral OCT system (RTVue XR Avanti, Optovue, Inc., Fremont, CA). Although the systems acquires fewer axial scans per second, high quality angiograms with more transverse points (304 × 304, **Fig. 1.2B**) are produced in less time (2.9 seconds). The higher performance is due to the lower decorrelation noise on the spectral OCT system, which requires only 2 consecutive cross-sectional scans at one position to compute a reliable decorrelation image. The higher transverse scan density, along with a higher transverse resolution associated with the shorter wavelength, means that the Avanti produces retinal angiograms with higher definition and higher resolution than the swept-source OCT prototype we originally used **(Figs 1.2C and D)**.

REFERENCES

1. Wang RK, et al. Three dimensional optical angiography. Opt Express. 2007;15:4083-97.
2. Grulkowski I, et al. Scanning protocols dedicated to smart velocity ranging in Spectral OCT. Opt Express. 2009;17:23736-54.
3. Yu L, Chen Z. Doppler variance imaging for three-dimensional retina and choroid angiography. J Biomed Opt. 2010;15:016029.
4. Makita S, Jaillon F, Yamanari M, Miura M, Yasuno Y. Comprehensive in vivo micro-vascular imaging of the human eye by dual-beam-scan Doppler optical coherence angiography. Optics Express. 2011;19:1271-83.
5. Zotter S, et al. Visualization of microvasculature by dual-beam phase-resolved Doppler optical coherence tomography. Optics Express. 2011;19:1217-27.
6. Braaf B, Vermeer KA, Vienola KV, de Boer JF. Angiography of the retina and the choroid with phase-resolved OCT using interval-optimized backstitched B-scans. Optics Express. 2012;20:20516-34.

7. Mariampillai A, et al. Speckle variance detection of microvasculature using swept-source optical coherence tomography. Opt Lett. 2008;33:1530-2.
8. Motaghiannezam R, Fraser S. Logarithmic intensity and speckle-based motion contrast methods for human retinal vasculature visualization using swept source optical coherence tomography. Biomed Opt Express. 2012;3:503-21.
9. Enfield J, Jonathan E, Leahy M. In vivo imaging of the microcirculation of the volar forearm using correlation mapping optical coherence tomography (cmOCT). Biomed Opt Express. 2011;2:1184-93.
10. Fingler J, Zawadzki RJ, Werner JS, Schwartz D, Fraser SE. Volumetric microvascular imaging of human retina using optical coherence tomography with a novel motion contrast technique. Opt Express. 2009;17:22190-200.
11. Liu G, Lin AJ, Tromberg BJ, Chen Z. A comparison of Doppler optical coherence tomography methods. Biomed Opt Express. 2012;3:2669-80.
12. Jia Y, et al. Split-spectrum amplitude-decorrelation angiography with optical coherence tomography. Opt Express. 2012;20:4710-25.
13. Tokayer J, Jia Y, Dhalla AH, Huang D. Blood flow velocity quantification using split-spectrum amplitude-decorrelation angiography with optical coherence tomography. Biomed Opt Express. 2013;4:1909-24, doi:10.1364/BOE.4.001909 193860 [pii].
14. Riva CE, Petrig B. Blue field entoptic phenomenon and blood velocity in the retinal capillaries. J Opt Soc Am. 1980;70:1234-8.
15. Tam J, Tiruveedhula P, Roorda A. Characterization of single-file flow through human retinal parafoveal capillaries using an adaptive optics scanning laser ophthalmoscope. Biomed Opt Express. 2011;2:781-93. doi:10.1364/BOE.2.000781.
16. Lopez-Saez M, et al. Fluorescein-induced allergic reaction. Annals of Allergy, Asthma and Immunology. 1998;81:428-30.
17. Hendargo HC, McNabb RP, Dhalla AH, Shepherd N, Izatt JA. Doppler velocity detection limitations in spectrometer-based versus swept-source optical coherence tomography. Biomed Opt Express. 2011;2:2175-88.
18. Blatter C, et al. Ultrahigh-speed non-invasive widefield angiography. Biomed Opt Express. 2012;17:0705051-3.

2 Interpretation of Optical Coherence Tomography Angiography

David Huang, Yali Jia, Simon S Gao

INTRODUCTION

This chapter refers to optical coherence tomography (OCT) angiography performed using the split-spectrum amplitude decorrelation angiography (SSADA) algorithm on either a swept-source OCT prototype or a commercial spectral OCT system (RTVue-XR Avanti, Optovue, Inc., Fremont, CA). But the generally principles are also applicable to other types of OCT angiography.

ANATOMIC REFERENCE PLANES AND ANGIOGRAPHIC SLABS

Optical coherence tomography (OCT) angiography produces three-dimensional (3D) flow data that requires segmentation into different layers to optimally evaluate abnormalities. Computer segmentation of OCT images provides the reference planes or surface. Appropriate tissue layers or "slabs" are then defined relative to these reference planes. The useful reference planes include the inner limiting membrane (ILM), outer boundary of the inner plexiform layer (IPL), outer boundary of the outer plexiform layer (OPL), and Bruch's membrane (BM). Automated algorithms perform well in identifying these reference planes in scans of healthy eyes. However, in cases where the retina is deformed, manual correction of the reference planes or adjustment of slab boundaries may be required.

Cross-sectional OCT angiograms combine color-coded decorrelation or flow information superimposed on gray-scale reflectance signal (Fig. 2.1A). Using this technique, both blood flow and retinal structural information are presented together. This is useful to provide detailed information on the depth of abnormalities such retinal or choroidal neovascularization.

En face presentation of OCT angiography helps clinicians recognize vascular patterns associated with various vascular abnormalities. *En face* angiograms are generated by summarizing the flow information within the depth range encompassed by relevant anatomic layers (slab), typically by taking the maximum or average decorrelation (representing flow) value. This projection process compresses the three-dimensional (3D) angiogram into several two-dimensional (2D) images that can be more easily interpreted. Using the segmentation of the ILM, outer boundary of the IPL, outer boundary of the OPL, retinal pigment epithelium (RPE), and BM, the following slabs can be visualized:

- *Vitreous*: Normally avascular (above the ILM)
- *Superficial retinal plexus*: Superficial portion of the inner retina (ILM to outer boundary of the IPL)
- *Deep retinal plexus*: Deep portion of the inner retina (outer boundary of the IPL to outer boundary of the OPL)
- *Inner retina*: The combination of superficial and deep retinal plexi (ILM to outer boundary of the OPL)
- *Outer retina*: Normally avascular (outer boundary of the OPL to RPE)
- *Choriocapillaris*: Normally near confluent (BM to 10–20 µm below)

Interpretation of Optical Coherence Tomography Angiography | 7

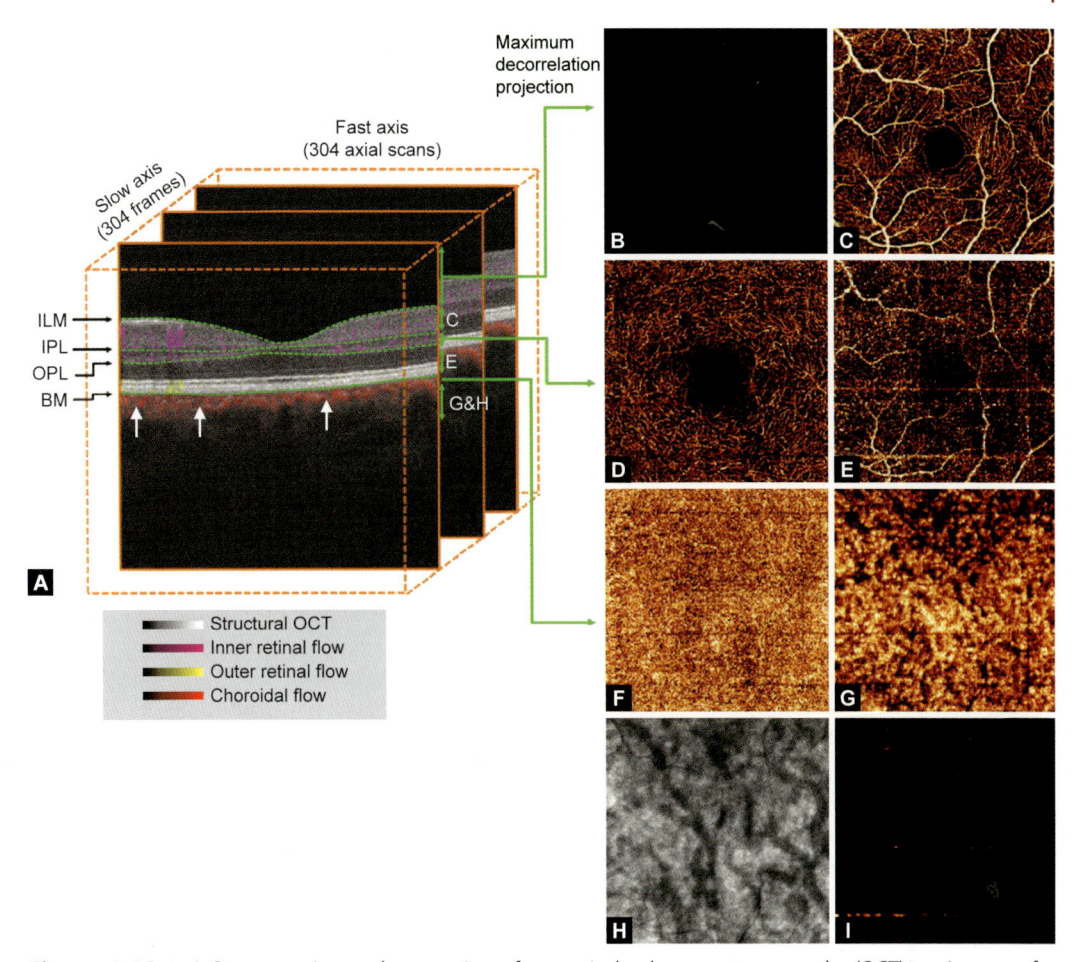

Figures 2.1A to I Segmentation and processing of an optical coherence tomography (OCT) angiogram of a normal macula. (A) The 3D-OCT angiogram comprises 304 frames of averaged decorrelation cross-sections stretched along the slow scan axis. Each frame is computed using the split-spectrum amplitude decorrelation angiography (SSADA) algorithm. The angiogram spans 3 mm in all 3 dimensions. The cross-sectional angiogram shows that flow in the inner retinal vessels (purple) are projected onto bright photoreceptor and retinal pigment epithelium (RPE) layers (indicated by white arrows). Image processing software separates the vitreous, inner retinal layers, outer retinal layers, and choroidal layers along the inner limiting membrane (ILM), outer boundary of the inner plexiform layer (IPL), outer boundary of the outer plexiform layer (OPL), and Bruch's membrane (BM) (dotted green lines). Six segmented flow volumes are separately projected. The projection algorithm finds the maximum decorrelation value for each transverse position within the segmented depth range, representing the fastest flowing vessel lumen in the segmented tissue layers; (B) *Vitreous*: The vitreous angiogram shows the absence of vascular flow; (C) *Superficial retinal plexus*: The superficial inner retinal angiogram shows normal retinal circulation with a small foveal avascular zone of approximately 0.6 mm in diameter; (D) *Deep retinal plexus*: The deep inner retina angiogram shows the deep retinal plexus which is a network of fine vessels: (E) *Outer retina*: The outer retina slab shows flow projection artifacts cast by flowing blood in the inner retinal vessels onto the RPE; (F) *Choriocapillaris*: The choriocapillaris angiogram; (G) *Deeper choroid*: The deeper choroid angiogram; (H) *Deeper choroid*: The deeper choroid *en face* structural OCT; (I) The outer retinal angiogram after removal of the projection artifact using a postprocessing algorithm

- *Deeper choroid*: Larger choroidal vessels (more than 20 µm below BM)
- *Choroid*: The combination of choriocapillaris and deeper choroid
- *Custom*: User defined slab that best highlight the vascular pathology.

In a healthy eye, an *en face* OCT angiogram above the ILM shows the normal, avascular vitreous (**Fig. 2.1B**). The inner retina shows larger vessels in the superficial plexus (**Fig. 2.1C**) and fine capillary network in the deep plexus (**Fig. 2.1D**) with no flow in the foveal avascular zone (FAZ). The outer retina should be avascular, but flow projection artifacts from the inner retina can be seen (**Fig. 2.1E**). The flow projection artifact occurs because flow blood in the retinal vessels cast flickering shadows that cause OCT signal fluctuation in the layers below that is recognized as flow by the OCT angiography algorithm. Amplitude/magnitude/intensity-based, phase-based and complex amplitude-based OCT angiography are all susceptible to similar flow projection artifacts. This shadowgraphic fluctuation is most noticeable in highly reflective layers such as the retinal pigment epithelium (RPE) and form a pattern that replicates the retinal circulation (**Fig. 2.1E**). The flow projection artifact can be suppressed by postprocessing software (**Fig. 2.1I**). The choriocapillaris shows nearly confluent flow (**Fig. 2.1F**). Although artifactual projection of retinal vessels in the choriocapillaris is present, it is not very noticeable because the artifact is diffused by the overlying RPE and weaker than the predominant choriocapillaris circulation. Lobular structures of the choriocapillaris are difficult to recognize because it is very dense within the macula and beyond the limited transverse spatial resolution. The coarser lobules outside the macula would be recognizable. The deeper choroid angiogram shows larger vessels but is more difficult to interpret due to flow projection, shadowing, and fringe-washout artifacts. Fringe washout occurs because high flow velocity (especially the axial component) mixes the phase of the interferometric signal within the integration time of the camera or photodetector in the OCT system.[1] Together with shadowing, fringe washout can reduce OCT signal intensity below that needed for SSADA processing. Therefore, part of or entire large choroidal vessels can appear dark on both *en face* OCT angiography (**Fig. 2.1G**) and structural OCT (**Fig. 2.1H**).

ANGIOVUE DEFAULT SEGMENTATION AND DISPLAY

AngioVue™ (Optovue, Inc., Fremont, CA) is currently the only OCT angiography software available on a commercially available high-speed (70 kHz axial scan repetition rate) OCT system (RTVue-XR Avanti). It uses the SSADA algorithm to detect flow, and an orthogonal registration algorithm called "Motion Correction Technology" (MCT) to remove motion artifacts. AngioVue provides a default angiographic display scheme that defines *en face* angiographic slabs relative to a simplified set of reference planes that can be reliably segmented by current software. These include the ILM, outer boundary of IPL, and the "RPE Reference," which is the best-fit surface under the retinal pigment epithelium and approximates the BM position. For the convenience of AngioVue users, the 4 default *en face* display slab definitions are provided here:

- *Superficial retinal capillary plexus*: 3 µm below the ILM to 15 µm below IPL
- *Deep retinal capillary plexus*: 15–70 µm below the IPL
- *Outer retina*: 70 µm below the IPL to 30 µm below the RPE Reference
- *Choroid capillary*: 30–60 µm below the RPE Reference.

These definitions are optimized for the detection of common pathologies using the automated segmentation algorithm within the AngioVue software. Therefore, they are at slight variance from the idealized layer boundaries we outlined in the last section. The automatically segmented reference planes could be manually corrected, and the slab border offset could be adjusted relative to the reference planes. With these flexibilities, the user could shift the slabs to highlight any pathology. The AngioVue outer retinal slab allows for suppression of flow projection artifact from the overlying retinal blood vessel onto the RPE. This can be turned on or off with a "Remove Artifacts" check box. Artifact suppression is useful for the clean visualization of choroidal neovascularization (CNV) and is explained in more detail further.

Recognizing Flow Projection Artifact and Nonvascular Flow Signal

Shadowgraphic flow projection artifacts result from fluctuating shadows cast by flowing blood in the large inner retinal vessels that cause variation of the OCT signal in deeper layers. Similarly, CNV component above BM could project onto choroidal layers below. This signal variation would be detected as a decorrelation and could not be differentiated from true flow based on signal characteristics alone. The clinician can recognize the flow projection artifact by noting that it forms a vertical streak in the cross-sectional OCT angiogram **(Fig. 2.1A)**, and that the vascular pattern of a more superficial layer is replicated on a deeper layer **(Fig. 2.1E compared to 2.1C)**. It is particularly important not to be fooled by this artifact in the detection of CNV. The RPE is the dominant screen on which the retinal blood flow is projected. This produces a prominent flow projection artifact in the outer retinal slab that is reduced using a projection artifact suppression algorithm in the AngioVue software **(Figs 2.2A to C)**. The algorithm still leaves residual patchy flow signal that are nonvascular in origin. This nonvascular flow signal is again most noticeable in highly scattering tissue (e.g. RPE). This artifact does not have the distinct patterns presented by CNV, which are described in the last section of this chapter. CNV is ruled out in this dry age-related macular degeneration (AMD) example by the absence of any distinct CNV vascular pattern in artifact-suppressed outer retina slab as well as the choriocapillaris slab.

Quantification: Flow Index and Vessel Density

The SSADA allows for the quantification of blood flow within the regions of interest. The flow index and vessel density can be determined from the *en face* maximum projection angiogram. The flow index is calculated as the average decorrelation value (which is correlated with flow velocity) in the selected region. The vessel density is calculated as the percentage area occupied by vessels and microvasculature in the selected region.

Typical Regions of Interest

For scans of the macula, flow index and vessel density can be routinely determined for the parafovea and/or perifovea. The parafovea is defined to be an annular region with an inner diameter of 0.6 mm and outer diameter of 2.5 mm centered on the FAZ. The perifovea is defined to be the annular region extending from the edge of the parafovea to an outer diameter of 5.5 mm. These zones are illustrated on a 6 × 6 mm macular retinal angiogram of a normal eye in **Figure 2.3B**.

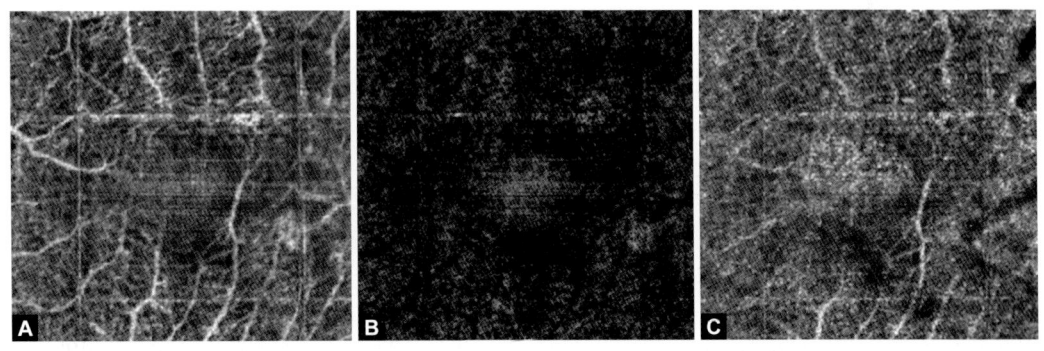

Figures 2.2A to C AngioVue OCT angiography of an eye with dry age-related macular degeneration: (A) *En face* OCT angiogram of the outer retina shows dense flow projection from the retinal vasculature above; (B) *En face* OCT angiogram of the outer retina after application of the projection artifact removal algorithm show residual patches of nonvascular flow signal. They can be recognized as artifact because they do not have any distinct vascular pattern; (C) *En face* OCT angiogram of the choriocapillaris does not show any choroidal neovascularization (CNV) pattern

10 | Practical Handbook of OCT Angiography

For scans of the optic nerve head, flow index and vessel density can be routinely determined for the peripapillary retina. The peripapillary is defined as an elliptical annulus extending outward from the optic disc boundary.

Interpretation of Pathological Optical Coherence Tomography Angiography

On OCT angiography, pathology is identified by the absence or reduction of flow in normally vascular layers or abnormal vascular patterns in normally avascular layers.

Detection of Capillary Dropout and Measurement of Nonperfusion Area

Optical coherence tomography (OCT) angiography can visualize areas of capillary dropout. In a normal eye **(Figs 2.3A to C)**, the retinal capillary network is dense with the exception of the FAZ, where capillaries are normally absent. In an eye with proliferative diabetic retinopathy **(Figs 2.4A to D)**, areas of nonperfusion could be identified outside of the FAZ using custom software.

Detection of Retinal Neovascularization

The development of retinal neovascularization (RNV) signifies progression to the proliferative case of diabetic retinopathy. The recognition of RNV is important as it may guide the treatment decision regarding panretinal photocoagulation which has been shown reduce the risk of vision loss due to RNV.[2] OCT angiography can be used to distinguish between intraretinal microvascular abnormalities, which occupy the same plane as the retinal blood vessels, and early RNV, which develops anterior to the ILM **(Figs 2.4A to D)**. The extent and activity of RNV can also be quantified on OCT angiography by flow index and vessel area. The commercial AngioVue software does not have a default vitreous slab currently, but the user could obtain such a view by manually shifting the superficial retinal plexus slab upward.

Detection of Choroidal Neovascularization

Choroidal neovascularization (CNV), the primary pathologic feature of neovascular AMD, consists of abnormal blood vessels growth from the choriocapillaris. The CNV penetrate through BM

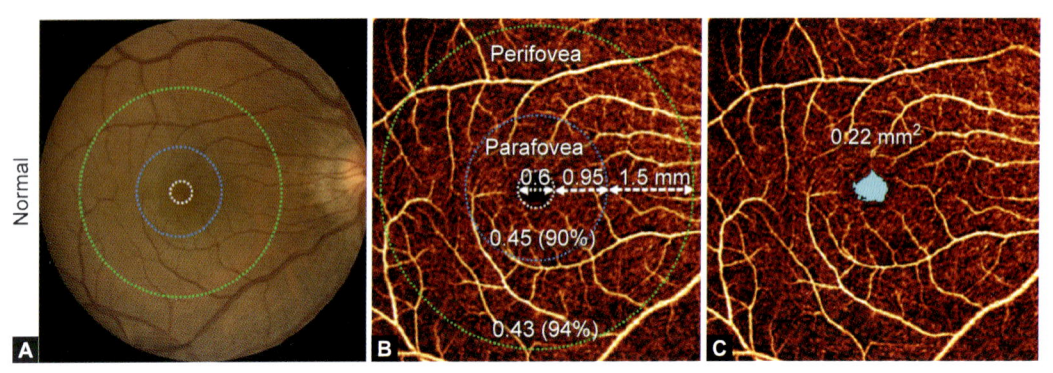

Figures 2.3A to C Quantification of inner retinal blood flows in a normal eye using OCT angiography acquired using the RTVue-XR OCT system. White dashed circle: normal foveal avascular zone (FAZ, 0.6 mm diameter white dashed circle). Area between white and blue dashed circles: parafoveal zone. Area between blue and green dashed circles: perifoveal zone. (A) Fundus photo; (B) *En face* 6 × 6 mm OCT angiogram of the inner retina. Parafoveal and perifoveal retinal flow indexes (vessel densities) were calculated using custom software; (C) An avascular area (blue) was identified in the normal FAZ with area of 0.22 mm² using a custom software developed by the authors

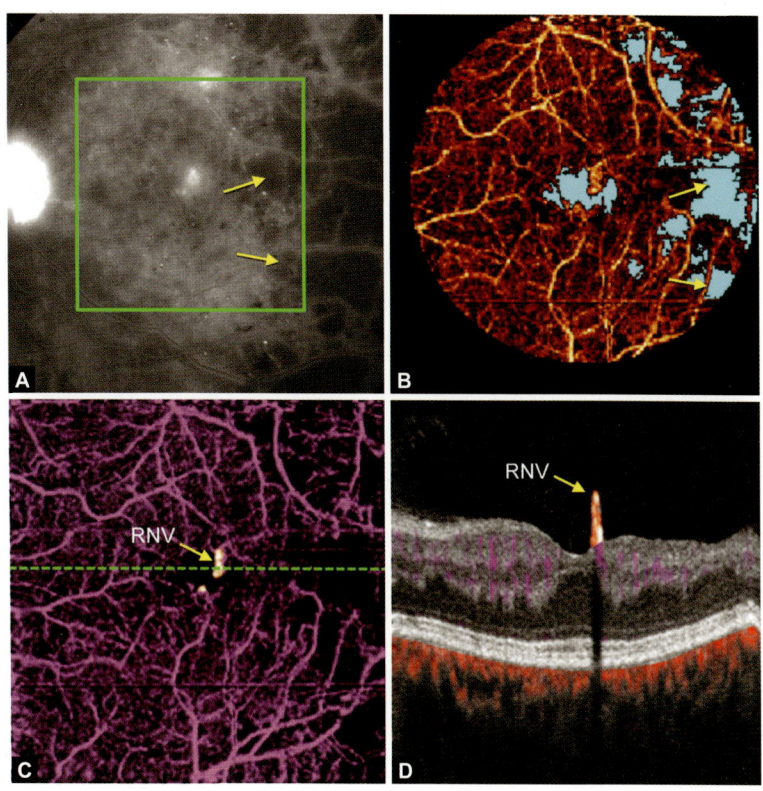

Figures 2.4A to D Proliferative diabetic retinopathy imaged using RTVue-XR AngioVue and processed with custom software. (A) Late frame fluorescein angiogram showing numerous microaneurysms, hyperfluorescence at the fovea, and regions of hypofluorescence temporal to the fovea (yellow arrows). The green square outlines the 6 × 6 mm area shown on the OCT angiogram; (B) Avascular areas (blue) were identified on the inner retinal *en face* OCT angiogram using custom software; (C) Composite *en face* OCT angiogram showing flow signal of retinal neovascularization (RNV, yellow) above the inner limit membrane (ILM) on a background of retinal vessels (purple); (D) Cross-sectional OCT angiogram RNV (yellow) above the ILM. Inner retinal flow is in purple; choroidal flow is in red
Abbreviation: RNV, retinal neovascularization

into the subretinal pigment epithelium (RPE) space and subretinal space. Subsequent exudation and hemorrhage damage retinal tissues, resulting in vision loss.[3] Detection and classification of CNV as Type I or II relies on proper segmentation. Examples using Optovue's AngioVue software are shown.

In an example of Type I CNV **(Figs 2.5A to C)**, absence of the CNV in the outer retinal slab above the RPE and presence of the CNV in the slab below the RPE establishes it as Type I. Because Type I CNV is below the RPE, it projects very well into the choroidal slab. Thus, the choroidal slab is an excellent view for Type I CNV detection. However, one must keep in mind that the CNV network visualized in the *en face* OCT angiogram of the choroidal slab includes a projected component that is above the BM, as well as the true choroidal component below the BM.

In an example of Type II CNV **(Figs 2.6A to C)**, the abnormal vessels are well visualized in the default AngioVue outer retinal slab. To determine whether the CNV has a component above the RPE, it is necessary to move the lower boundary of the slab above the RPE to see if the CNV can still be visualized. In this case, much of the CNV

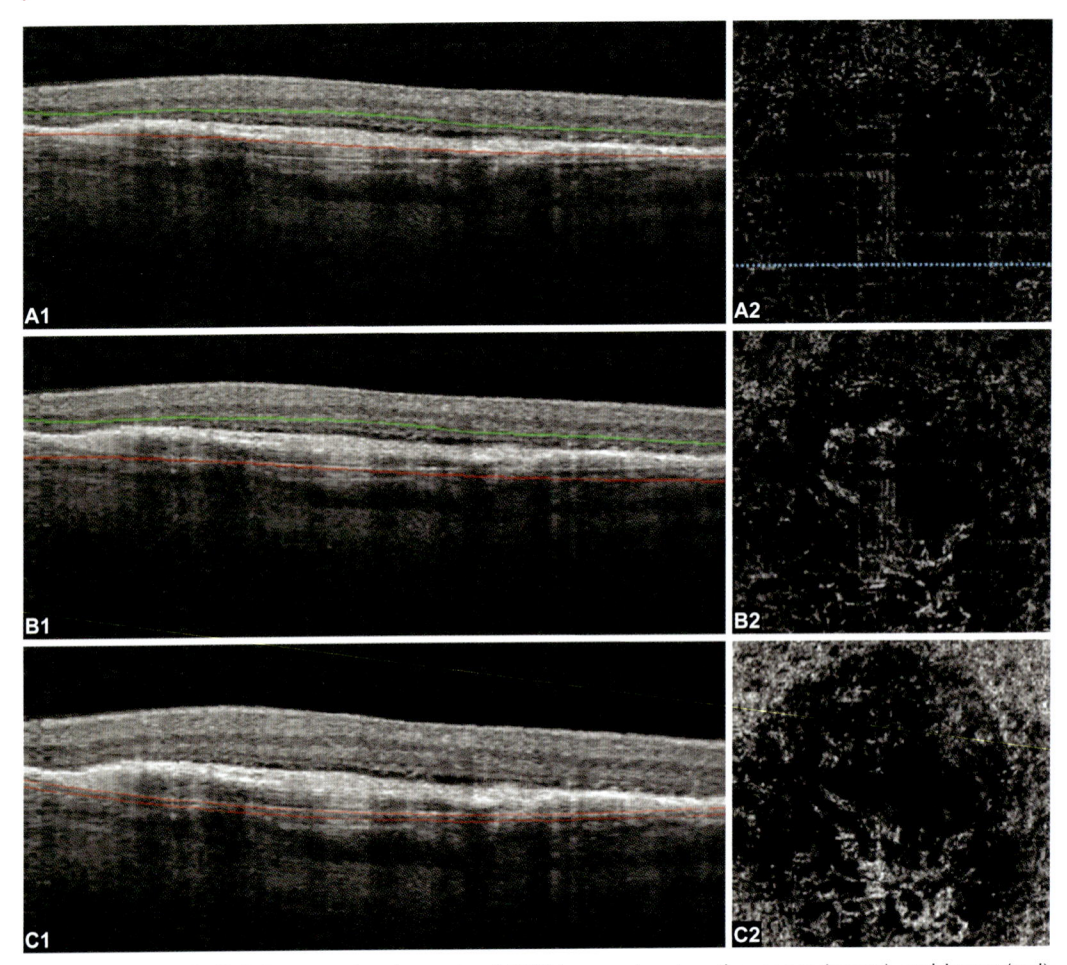

Figures 2.5A to C (A1) Cross-sectional structural OCT image showing the upper (green) and lower (red) boundaries of the outer retinal slab as defined by the default AngioVue software segmentation. It includes the RPE and above, (A2) *En face* angiogram of the outer retina as defined by the segmentation in (A1) showing no CNV. The blue dotted line shows the location of (A1); (B1) The same structural image with the lower boundary of the slab moved 100 μm lower to the level of the BM, (B2) The resulting angiogram reveals the presence of Type I CNV. The AngioVue software was set to remove flow projection artifacts from these angiograms of the outer retinal slab; (C1) Cross-sectional structural OCT showing the borders of the choroidal slab at 30 and 60 μm below a manually corrected RPE Reference, (C2) *En face* OCT angiogram of the choroidal slab shows the CNV well

vessel pattern remains, thus classifying this case as Type II CNV. Note that the CNV pattern appears brighter in the choroidal slab because it was not filtered by the artifact removal algorithm. But the CNV patterns appears the same both in the inner retinal slab and the choroidal slab, indicating that the CNV pattern in the choroid mostly represents projection from CNV above the BM, and not a large CNV component below the BM. Also note a dark shroud surrounding the CNV in the choroidal slab in both examples of Type I **(Figs 2.5A to C)** and Type II **(Figs 2.6A to C)** CNV. This is a common appearance that might indicate choroid defect in the region of the CNV.

Interpretation of Optical Coherence Tomography Angiography | 13

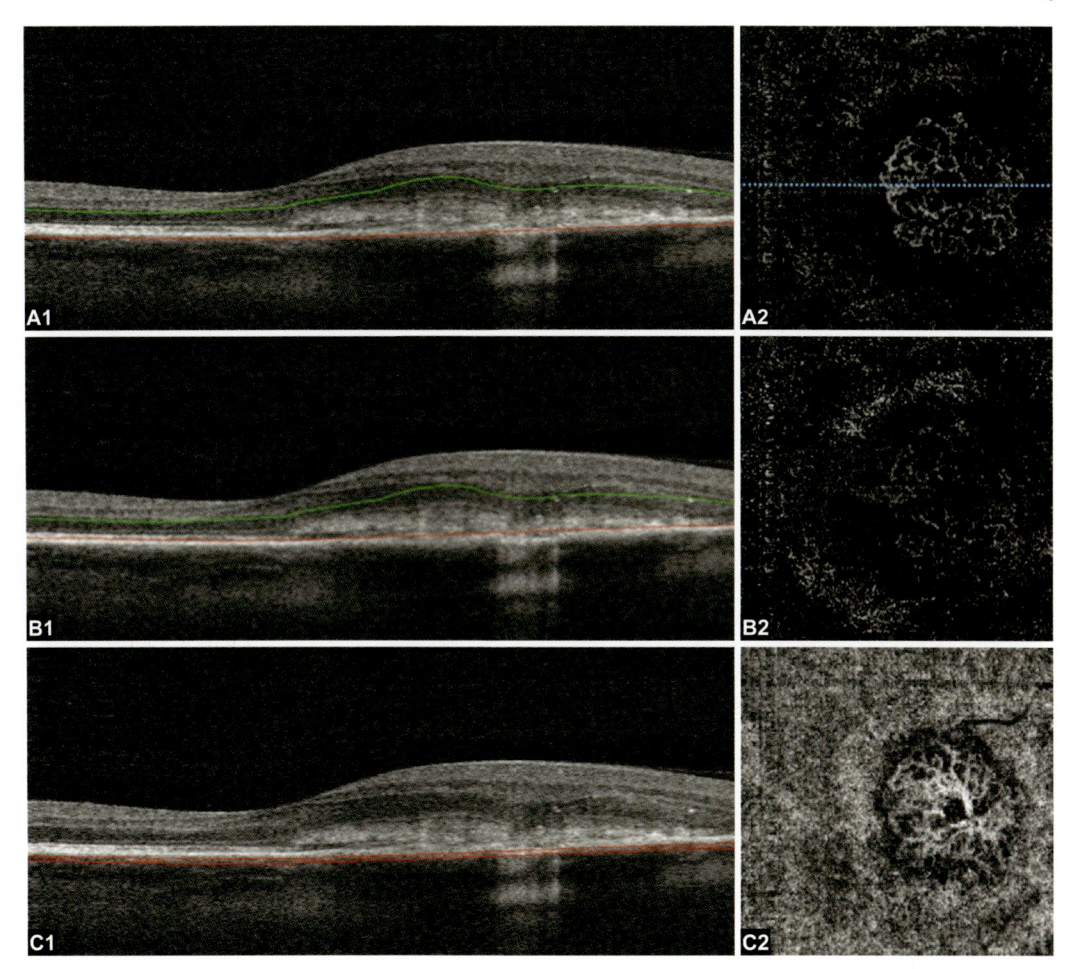

Figures 2.6A to C (A1) Cross-sectional structural OCT image showing the upper (green) and lower (red) boundaries of the outer retina slab as defined by the default AngioVue software segmentation, (A2) *En face* angiogram of the outer retinal slab reveals CNV. The blue dotted line shows the location of (A1); (B1) The same structural image with the lower boundary of the outer retinal slab adjusted 47 μm upward to a level just above the RPE, (B2) The resulting angiogram shows that the CNV exists above the RPE. The AngioVue software was set to remove flow projection artifacts from these angiograms of the outer retinal slab; (C1) Cross-sectional structural OCT showing the borders of the choroidal slab at 30 and 60 μm below RPE Reference, (C2) *En face* OCT angiogram of the choroidal slab clearly shows the CNV

Because retinal flow projection onto the outer retina slab can make it difficult to identify CNV, a color composite scheme can be used to aid in visualization **(Figs 2.7A to I)**.[4] In this example, a composite *en face* angiogram **(Fig. 2.7H)** shows the superficial retinal circulation **(Fig. 2.7D)** in purple and the outer retinal flow **(Fig. 2.7E)** in yellow. Areas of subretinal fluid are also shown in blue. Displaying the volumetric flow information as a composite image is advantageous as the retinal circulation in purple would mask the flow projection seen in the outer retina. In addition, it allows for identification of the CNV relative to landmarks in the superficial retinal vasculature.

14 | Practical Handbook of OCT Angiography

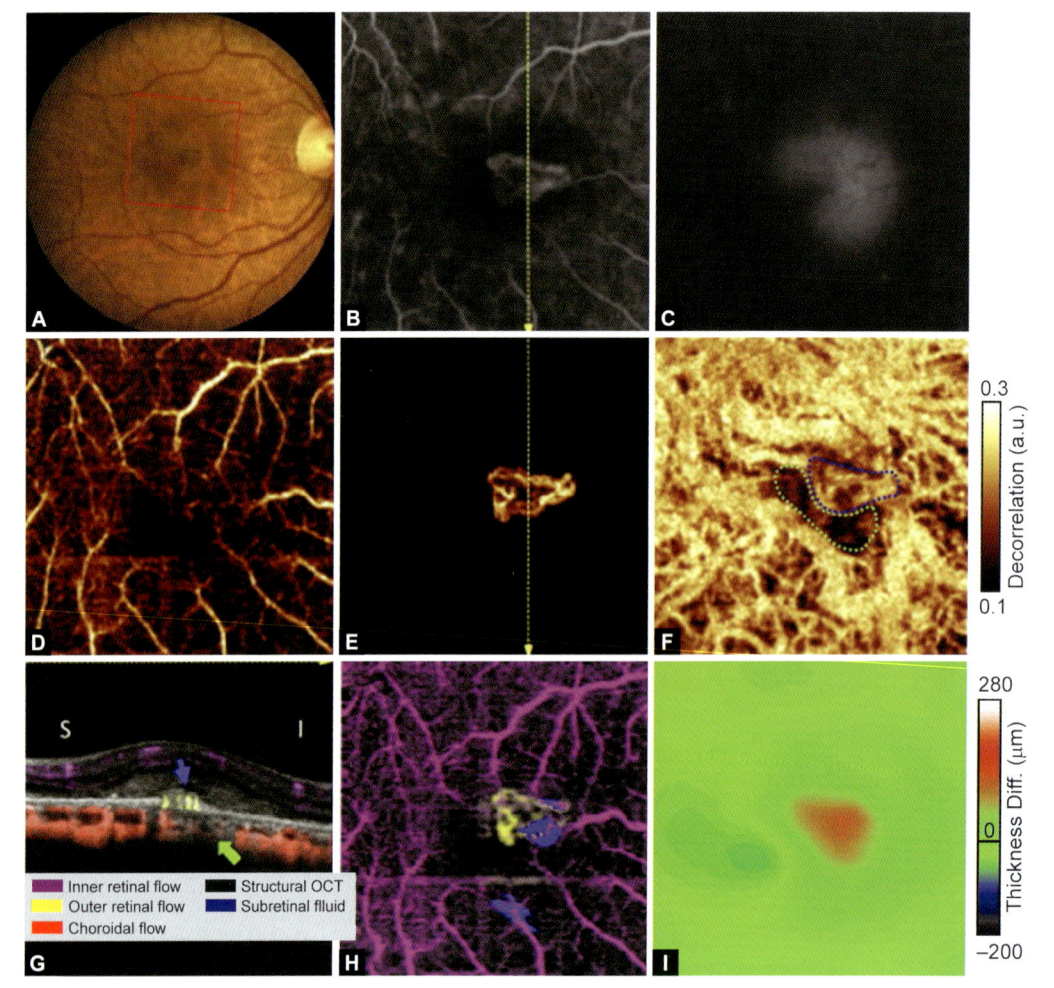

Figures 2.7A to I AMD patient with Type I choroidal neovascularization (CNV). (A) Color fundus photograph showing subretinal hemorrhage. Red square outlines the area shown on angiograms below; (B) Early-phase fluorescein angiography (FA); (C) Late-phase FA; (D) *En face* optical coherence tomography (OCT) angiogram of the inner retina; (E) *En face* angiogram of the outer retina showing the CNV. The *yellow dashed lines* indicate the position of OCT cross-section shown in (G). *Yellow arrows* indicate the superior to inferior direction; (F) *En face* angiogram of the choroid showing patchy flow directly under the CNV (*blue dotted outline*) and an adjacent area of reduced flow (*green dotted outline*); (G) Cross-sectional color OCT angiogram showing the CNV (*yellow*) was predominantly under the retinal pigment epithelial (RPE). The *blue arrow* shows the location of the subretinal fluid. The *green arrow* corresponds to the *green dashed outline* in (F) showing a focal region of reduced choroidal flow adjacent to the CNV; (H) Composite *en face* OCT angiograms showing most subretinal fluid (*dark blue*) inferior to the CNV; (I) Retinal thickness deviation map showing retinal thickening over the CNV

Abbreviations: I, inferior; S, superior, OCT, optical coherence tomography
Source: From reference 4

REFERENCES

1. Hendargo HC, McNabb RP, Dhalla AH, Shepherd N, Izatt JA. Doppler velocity detection limitations in spectrometer-based versus swept-source optical coherence tomography. Biomedical Optics Express. 2011;2:2175-88.
2. Group DRS R. Photocoagulation treatment of proliferative diabetic retinopathy: Clinical application of Diabetic Retinopathy Study (DRS) findings, DRS report number 8. Ophthalmology. 1981;88:583-600.
3. Ambati J, Ambati BK, Yoo SH, Ianchulev S, Adamis AP. Age-related macular degeneration: etiology, pathogenesis, and therapeutic strategies. Survey of Ophthalmology. 2003;48:257-93, doi:10.1016/s0039-6257(03)00030-4.
4. Jia Y, et al. Quantitative optical coherence tomography angiography of choroidal neovascularization in age-related macular degeneration. Ophthalmology. 2014;121(7):1435-44. doi:10.1016/j.ophtha.2014.01.034, S0161-6420(14)00104-3 [pii] (2014).

3A Quantification of Vascular Layers with Optical Coherence Tomography Angiography

Marco Rispoli

INTRODUCTION

The contribution of optical coherence tomography (OCT) angiography in visualizing the retinal microvasculature has been described extensively, and validated in routine clinical practice. Further, Angioanalytics, the recently developed software, enables addition of quantitative data to OCT angiography. Quantitative data, here, refers to a series of parameters that can be measured in the functional cube in a repeatable and reliable manner.

The parameters considered so far, and that are subject to further development, concern the flow area, the non-flow area, and the flow density area.

FLOW AREA

This type of measurement is of greatest interest in the follow-up of neovascular membranes, in particular, in the cases treated with intravitreal injections of anti-VEGF (vascular endothelial growth factors) or steroids. It is also important in the study of preretinal and prepapillary new vessel regression in proliferative retinopathies secondary to diabetes and venous occlusion. Unlike traditional fluorescein angiography, where staining and leakage of the dye tends to conceal the morphology of the neovascular network, OCT angiography does not track dye dynamics and only demonstrates the flows in the vascular structures of the segmented volume.

The measurement instrument requires the operator to trace the outline of the neovascular membrane after selecting the appropriate volume and segmentation profile (**Fig. 3A.1**). The software automatically identifies the outlined area and calculates the flow area. It is also possible to save the measurements for comparison at subsequent follow-up examination (**Fig. 3A.2**).

NONFLOW AREA (VASCULAR DROPOUT AREA)

The nonflow area is an area of ischemia or of vascular "dropout". The possibility of highlighting and comparing the nonflow areas applies to ischemic retinopathies. The nonflow areas are regions where there is no detectable flow by split-spectrum amplitude decorrelation angiography (SSADA). This tool seems to be useful in all ischemic retinopathies irrespective of the etiology. With OCT angiography, it is possible to separate nonflow areas at the superficial vascular plexus as well as at the deep vascular plexus.

After selecting the appropriate volume, on manually indicating any point in the nonflow area, the software automatically delimits the area that contains pixels having the same value (**Figs 3A.3A and B**). After proper *en face* projection, the software enables demonstration of nonperfused areas by mouse click selection. Ischemic areas are depicted in yellow, and may be saved and matched with other areas in the study. Data can be selected and saved for comparison with subsequent examinations.

FLOW DENSITY MAP

This instrument, made available recently, is designed for distinguishing flow areas from nonflow areas. The ratio of flow areas to nonflow areas

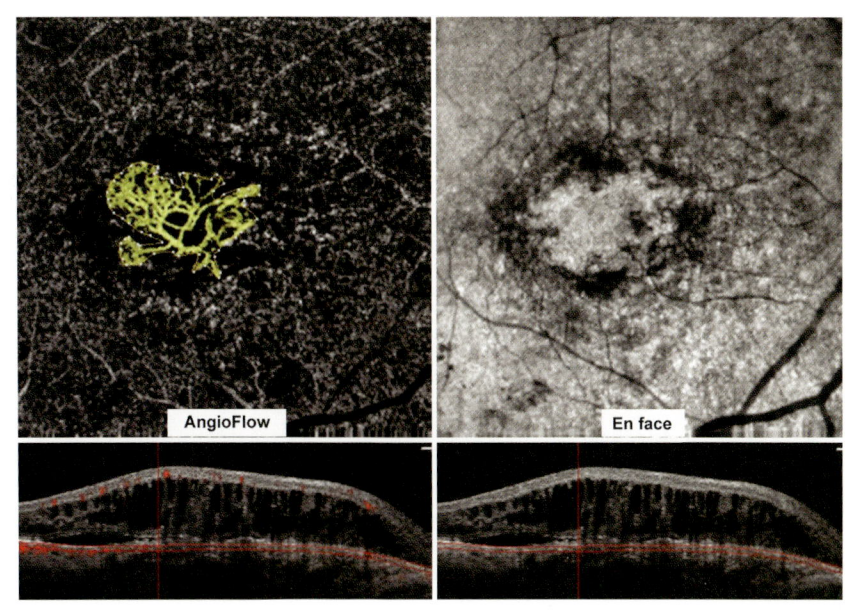

Quantification of Vascular Layers with Optical Coherence Tomography Angiography | **17**

Figure 3A.1 The neovascular membrane is marked by a dashed line and the flow in the new vessels appears in yellow. In the lower part of this image, the value of the area outlined by the operator appears alongside the value of the neovascular yellow area

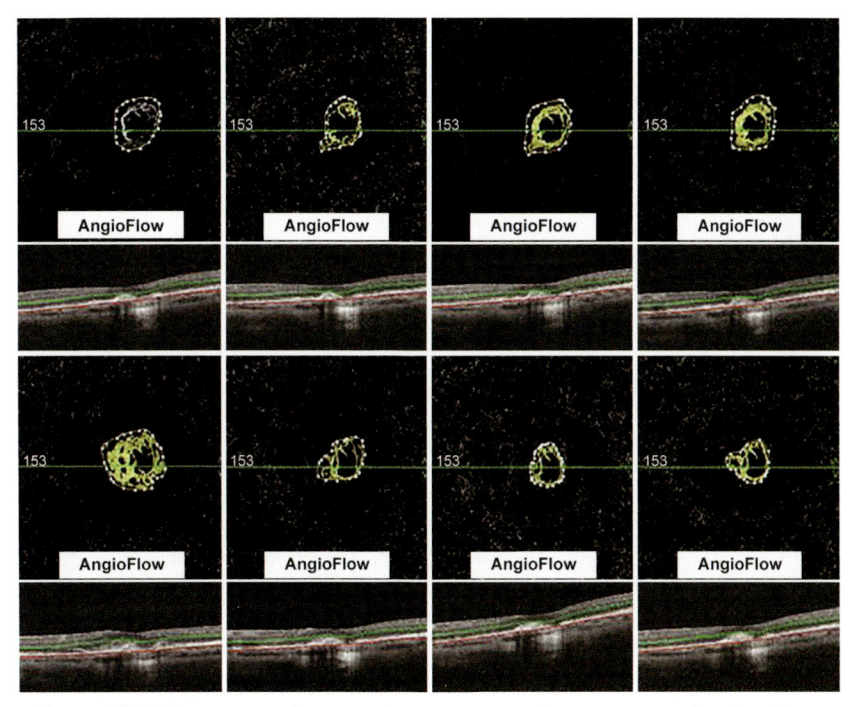

Figure 3A.2 The neovascular area measurement made at every examination allows for an immediate qualitative and numerical comparison

18 Practical Handbook of OCT Angiography

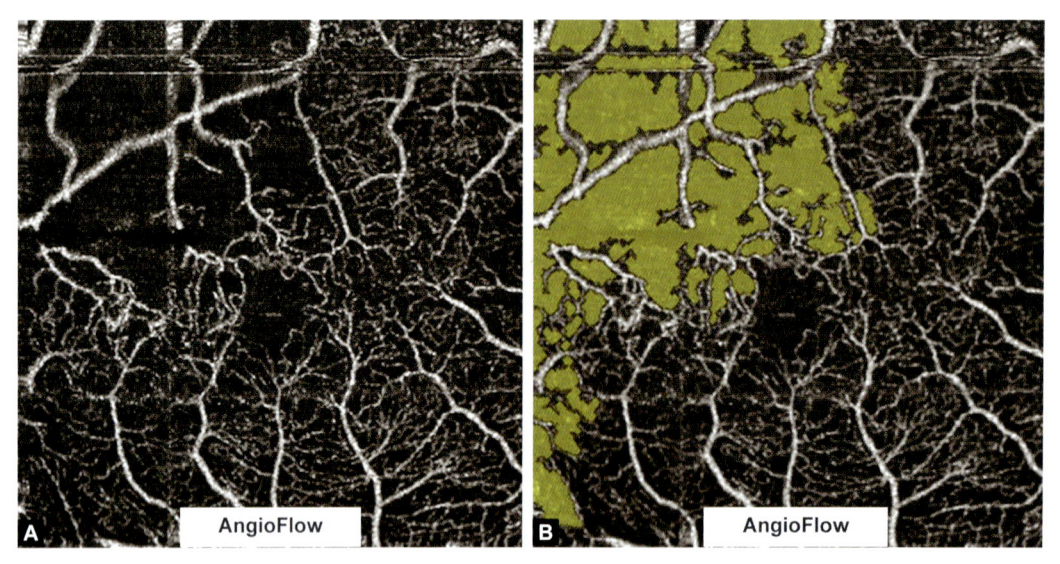

Figures 3A.3A and B (A) Venous occlusion of a branch with vascular dropout in the superficial vascular plexus; (B) The nonflow areas are highlighted in yellow, measured in mm^2, and compared with subsequent examinations

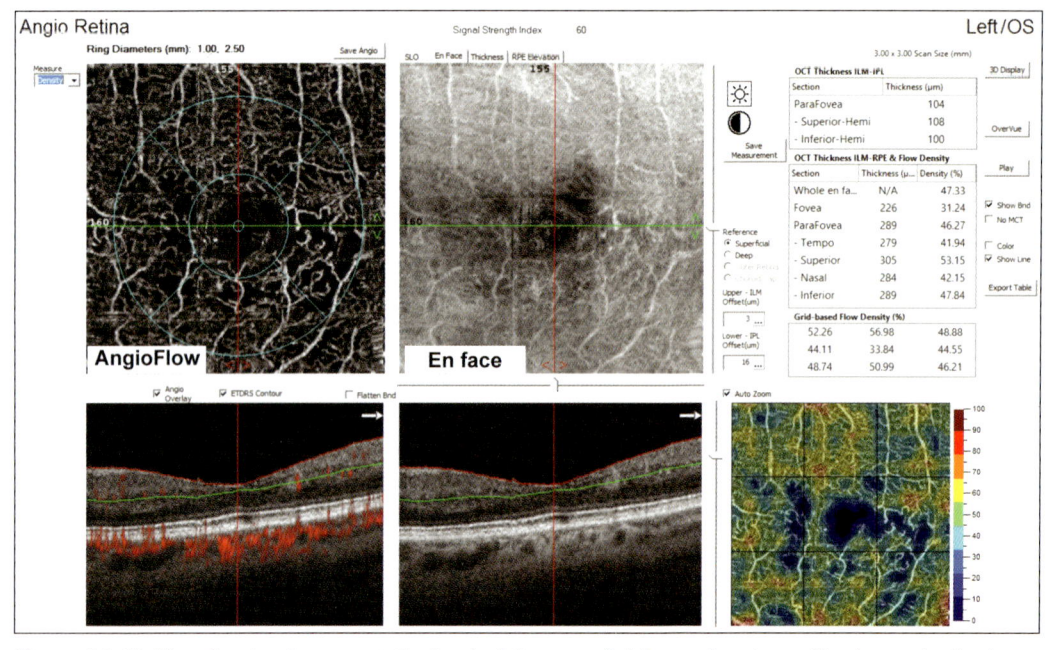

Figure 3A.4A Vascular density map at the level of the superficial vascular plexus. The image in the lower right shows a map of vascular density relative to the AngioFlow image in the upper left. The numerical values expressed in the upper right table refer to the circular grid superimposed onto the AngioFlow image

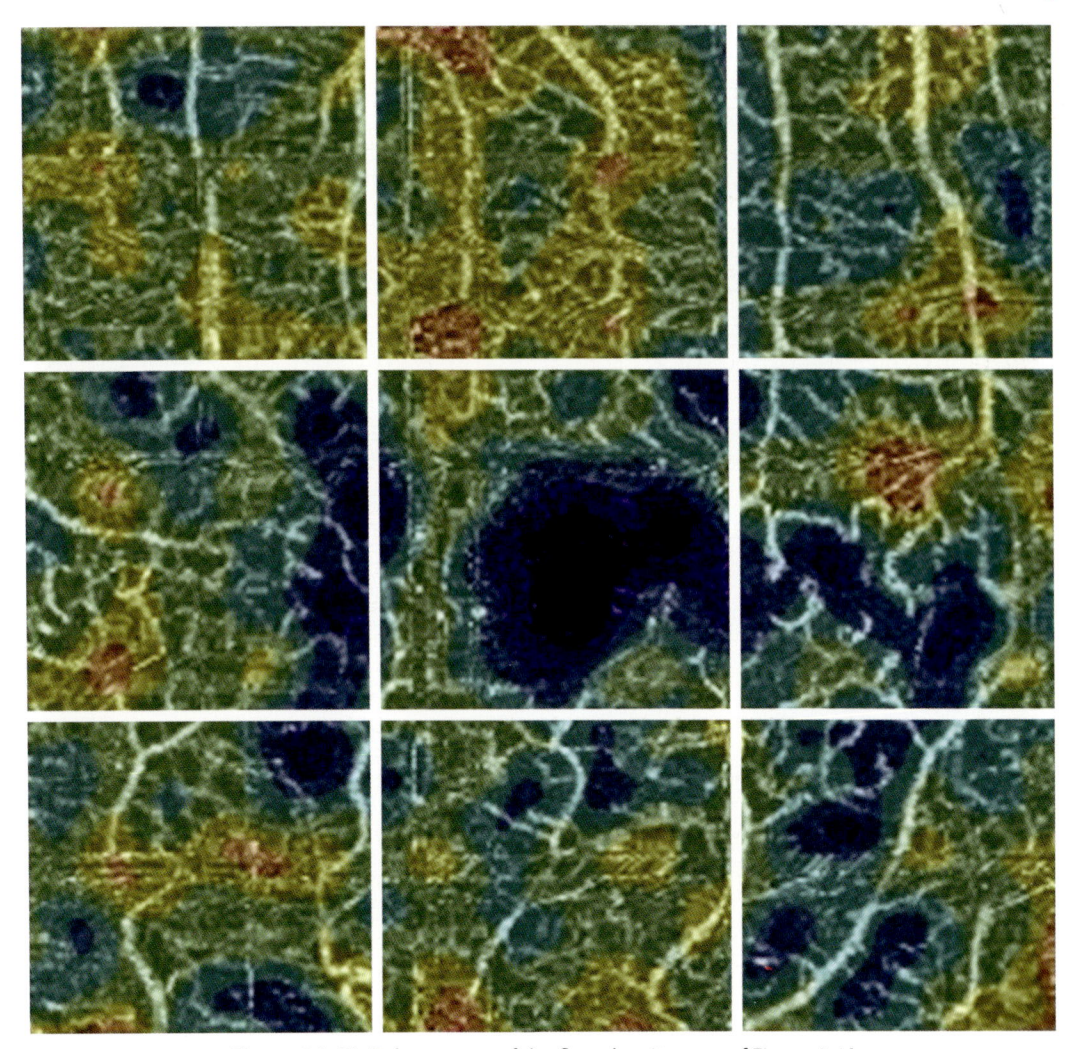

Figure 3A.4B Enlargement of the flow density map of Figure 3.4A

is expressed numerically as well as on a scale of false colors wherein warm colors are attributed to high flow density and cold colors are attributed to low flow density or absent density. The flow density map enables measurement of vascular area percentages on *en face* angiograms. This analysis is based on an Early Treatment Diabetic Retinopathy Study (ETDRS) grid centered on the macula as with the thickness map, thus providing an average vascular density value for each sector. The vascular density calculation may be applied to the volumetric scan of the superficial vascular plexus as well as the deep vascular plexus **(Figs 3A.4 and 3A.5)**.

20 Practical Handbook of OCT Angiography

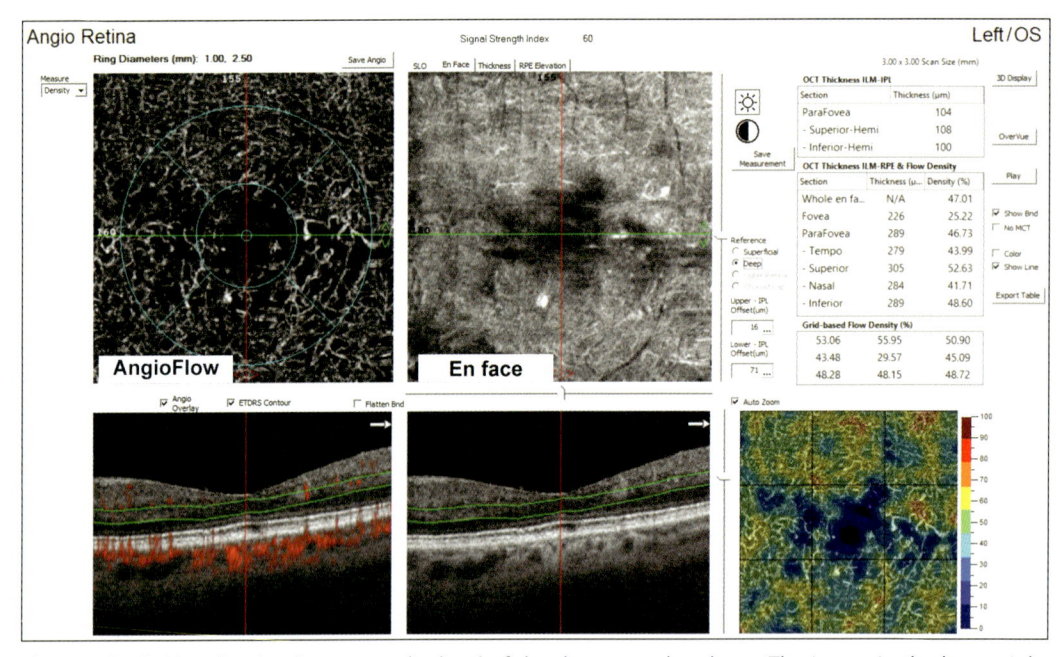

Figure 3A.5A Vascular density map at the level of the deep vascular plexus. The image in the lower right shows a map of vascular density relative to the AngioFlow image in the upper left. The numerical values expressed in the upper right table refer to the grid superimposed onto the AngioFlow image

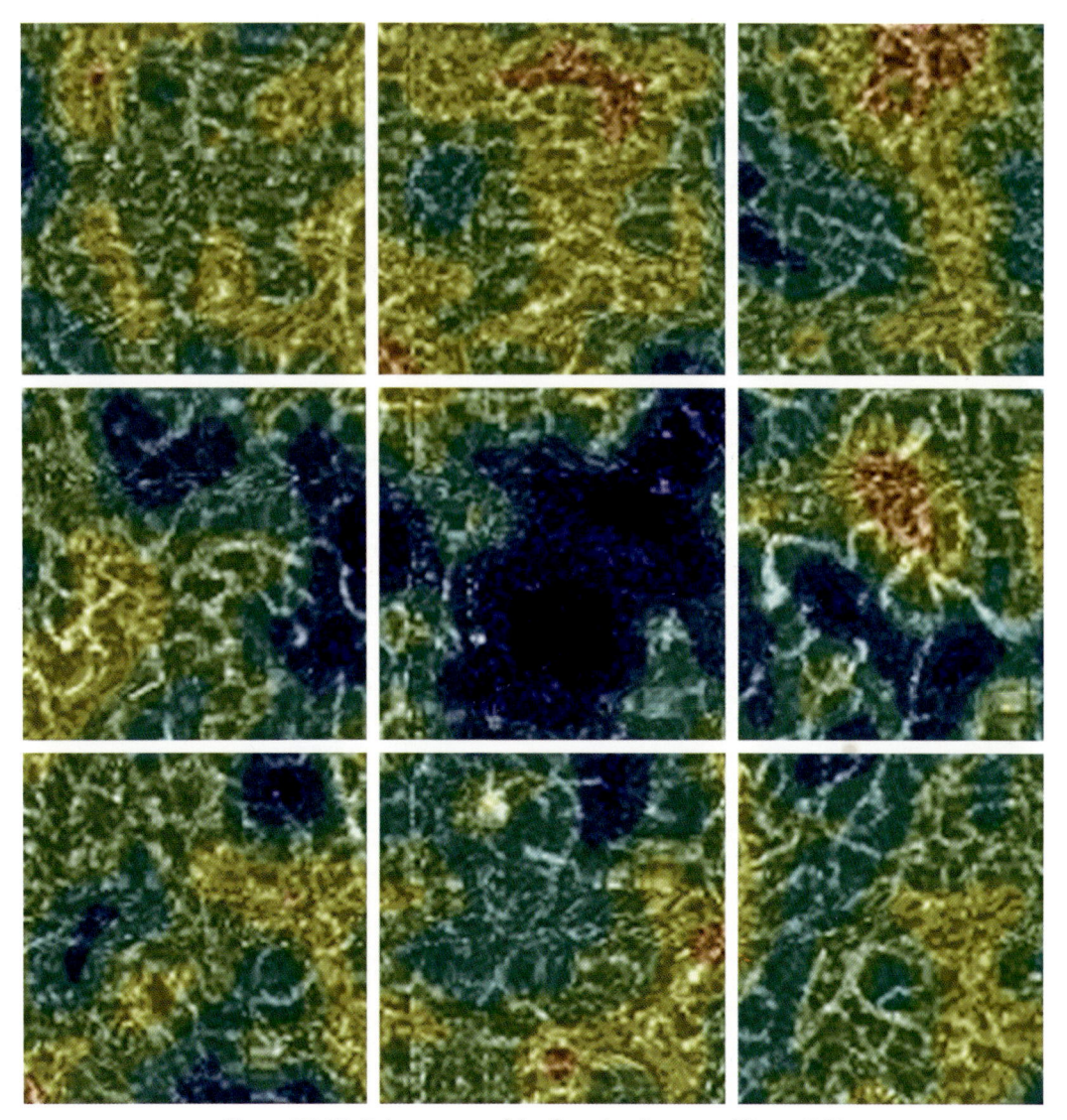

Figure 3A.5B Enlargement of the flow density map of Figure 3.5A

This instrument, whose repeatability is still under study, is potentially useful for the follow-up of diabetic retinopathies that are negative on ophthalmoscopy as well as in their more advanced stages. It is also likely to be useful in venous and arterial occlusion.

3B Practical Problems and Artifacts in Optical Coherence Tomography Angiography

Marco Rispoli, Bruno Lumbroso

Like all instrumental and imaging diagnostic examinations, the obtained results contain data directly related to the tissue being imaged, but also contain distortions or extraneous data that as a group are called artifacts. It is necessary to have a thorough knowledge of artifacts because they can provide false and misleading information.

Artifacts are common and originate in relation to image acquisition, intrinsic ocular characteristics, eye motion, image processing and display strategies. Each of these main classes of artifacts produces characteristic and recognizable image abnormalities.

Richard Spaide, James Fujimoto, Nadia Waheed[1] have classified and defined the artefacts and we hereby follow their indications:

Although there are a large number of potential artifacts the main artifacts commonly present are:
- *Movement artifacts*: Motion control software or similar techniques can alter the acquired image to reduce the effects of eye motion. Many instrument manufacturers are moving to eye tracking systems to avoid the problem in the first place. At present there are several consequences of eye movement:
  - *White line artifacts*: With eye movement during an image frame one region is imaged and is then juxtaposed with a noncontiguous region because of the movement. At the interface is a region with high decorrelation, which is rendered white. As a consequence this type of movement artifact is called a "white line artifact".
  - *Quilting defect*: The checkerboard defect or quilting defect occurs when the two horizontal and vertical raster sequences are quite different from one another due to eye movements and of saccades during the acquisition of each but the motion control software forces then to show alignment.
  - *Stretch artefact*: This is due to two images that are not exactly of the same region being combined and results in an area, typically at the edge of the image to be stretched or smeared in appearance. Stretch artifact can result from eye movement as well.
  - *Vessel doubling*: This is a problem linked to the MCT (motion correction technology) alignment system that cause some vessels to be seen doubled, side by side.
  - *Gap defect*: While the motion control software can reposition segments of the image to align more accurately with some eye movements there is going to be missing information. The missing information can appear as a gap in a blood vessel.
- *False negative flow*: Observed when flow is too slow and is below the detection threshold of the system, or the signal is attenuated by the opacities in the dioptric media or in the structures having a high scatter, like the retinal pigmented epithelium. Absence of flow signal does not necessarily mean there is a lack of vessels or factual flow. Therefore, the term flow void is used to describe the lack of visible flow within a region.
- *False positive flow (noflow areas)*: These are flows produced by the noise of eye movement. There are many sources of this error and this error is not corrected in current software.

These artifacts may fool vessel density and flow measurements to give artificially large measurements of each. Possible sources of false positive flow include: hard exudates, pigment accumulation, thrombosed microaneurysms or retinal hemorrhages and the borders of cystoid spaces. These artifacts need to be taken into account in order not to confuse nonvascular reflectivity with flow signals.

- *Projection artefact*: An important limitation of any motion contrast system is the perception that flow is occurring at levels other than the original vessels are located. Inner retinal vessels filter the light passing through them and with motion contrast processing may cause the appearance of the same vessels at the level of the retinal pigment epithelium (RPE). It is likely that mathematical correction can be performed to reduce projection artifacts, but the current methods used are primitive and cancel too much of the flow signal from deeper layers.
- *Saturation*: To be sensitive OCT angiography renders relatively small motion within a vessel as white and any increase in blood flow velocity is not rendered brighter as the image is white already. This strategy shows small low flow vessels, but does not provide visual feedback of the actual flow in vessels. Thus, the brightness of the vessel is said to saturate at low flow velocities. We know that blood flow in small vessels is lower than large vessels, but the image of each will be white.
- *Segmentation errors*: *En face* imaging depends on selecting particular layers of the retina to examine the contained vessels. In healthy tissue it is common to be able to accurately select specific layers and view the contained vessels. With diseased tissue or alterations from normal the algorithms used often fail. In normal eyes, the segmentation algorithms may show minor errors in one or more layers. Any deviation for normality increases the risk of segmentation error. In diabetic macular edema some layers may be greatly thickened, however the current segmentation strategies try to select layers with the same thickness as found in healthy eyes. This means the selected areas do not incorporate all of the necessary tissue and therefore, do not provide an accurate evaluation of blood flow. On the other hand, some retinal diseases cause the retina to become much thinner, and selection of standard thickness layers results in too much tissue being selected. High myopes have distortions of the ocular tissue and it is very common for segmentation algorithms to make many errors. Observation of a vascular layer as shown by OCT angiography without seeing the segmentation of the OCT imaging is usually not sufficient or trustworthy. There is no way to be certain of the accuracy of the selected slab position without seeing the evidence.

REFERENCE

1. Spaide RF, Fujimoto JG, Waheed NK. Image artefacts in optical coherence tomography angiography. Retina. 2015;35(11):2163-80.

4 Optical Coherence Tomography Angiography of Normal Retina and its Vascular Structure

Maria Cristina Savastano, Marco Rispoli, Bruno Lumbroso

INTRODUCTION

Optical coherence tomography (OCT) angiography shows the vascular structure of the retina *in vivo* without contrast agent. OCT angiography detects endoluminal flow at any time and is thus, independent of the time of administration of the contrast medium as in fluorescein angiography. However, at present, the periphery beyond the arches cannot yet be examined.

The classical anatomic studies described in the first half of the 20th century demonstrate the distribution of retinal vessels as organized into three distinct layers: (1) superficial plexus, observable with the ophthalmoscope, with the large and average sized vessels distributed in the retinal nerve fiber layer; (2) inner plexus, a body of small-sized capillaries located close to the inner surface of the inner nuclear layer; and (3) outer plexus: morphologically similar to the inner plexus but located on the outer surface of the outer plexiform layer.

OCT angiography has confirmed the findings of these studies *in vivo* and facilitates the separate study of the two vascular plexuses, the superficial vascular plexus and the internal/external that we consider as a single deep plexus. These two plexuses clearly have different features that cannot be distinguished by classical fluorescein angiography.

RETINAL VASCULAR NETWORKS

There are three vascular networks in the retina: one superficial and two deep. The resolution provided by OCT angiography with the split-spectrum amplitude-decorrelation angiography (SSADA) algorithm enables clear visualization of the superficial vascular plexus with a 60-micron section at the inner limiting membrane (ILM). The two deep plexuses cannot be clearly differentiated, since the smaller of 30-micron structures do not have sufficient resolution for them to be clinically useful. These two deep plexuses will therefore, be treated in this chapter as a single vascular entity, included in segmentation at the inner plexiform layer (IPL) of at least 30 microns.

The superficial vascular plexus is located in the ganglion cell layer and in the nerve fiber layer.

The two deep vascular nets are treated in this chapter as a single entity. They are located in the inner nuclear layers and external plexiform layer. From the anatomical standpoint, this plexus consists of two plexuses located respectively on the inside of the inner nuclear and on the outside of the outer plexiform layer. Since they cannot be individually seen by OCT angiography, they are considered as a single plexus.

In order to study the two main vascular plexuses, specific parameters that concern the intraretinal level (ILM, IPL, RPE , RPE ref), the thickness of the scan being examined and the offset are used. The need to establish very precise points of reference to analyze the vascular plexuses is determined in order to compare the analyses made by different operators and hence make the images as objective as possible.

The assessment of the superficial plexus (SP) uses a thickness of 60 μm from the ILM so as to include all the vessels of this plexus (**Fig. 4.1**). The parameters for the deep plexus (DP) are defined with reference to the IPL in a 30 μm thick

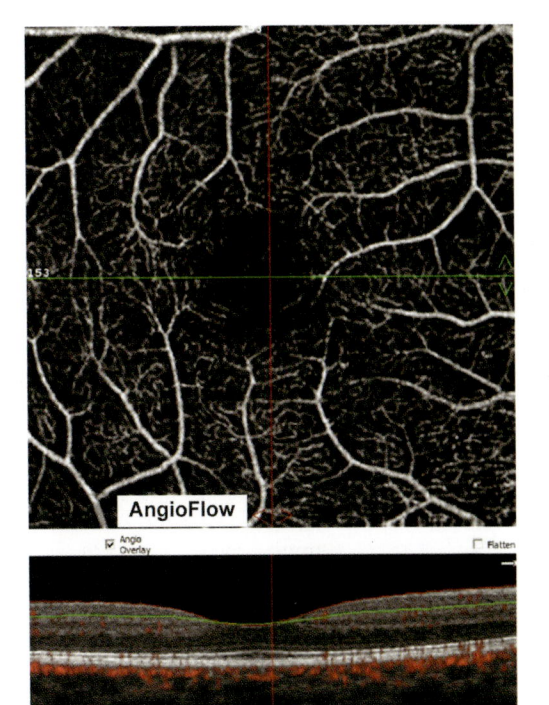

Optical Coherence Tomography Angiography of Normal Retina and its Vascular Structure | 25

Figure 4.1 *The superficial plexus:* There are multiple white linear structures (flow) against a black background that converge towards the fovea with a centripetal pattern. Secondary vessels leave the main vessels forming a spider web. Around the avascular area, the capillaries form continuous perifoveal arcades with regular meshes. Below, the B-scan shows normal vessels in red

Figure 4.2 *The deep plexus*: This consists of a close-knit pattern of vessels whose orderly distribution around the avascular foveal zone presents numerous thin horizontal and radial interconnections. The vessels fan out and interconnect to form a complex pattern. Below, the B-scan shows normal vessels in red

scan to visualize the deep plexus in its entirety (**Fig. 4.2**).

OCT angiography shows different morphological features of the retinal blood supply for the two plexuses considered.

The superficial plexus: The vascular distribution is represented by multiple white linear structures (flow) against a black background that converge towards the fovea with a centripetal pattern and originate from the large upper and lower vascular arcades. Secondary vessels leave the main vessels, forming a spider web. The thickness of the vessels is homogeneous throughout the length of the scan. The course of the vessels is always rather linear; the web is regular without sudden changes in direction or without vascular meanders or loops.

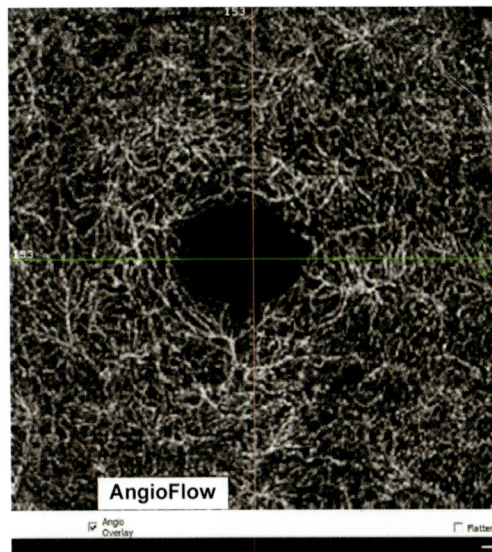

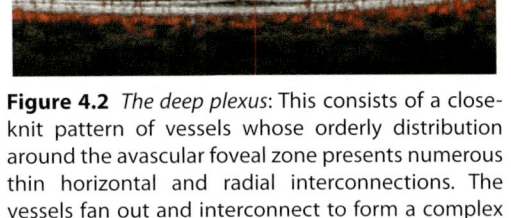

The vessels show a vascular signal (de-correlation) throughout the scan. Around the avascular area, the capillaries form continuous perifoveal arcades with regular meshes.

The deep plexus: This consists of a close-knit pattern of vessels whose orderly distribution around the avascular foveal zone presents numerous thin horizontal and radial interconnections. The pattern is concentric around the avascular foveal zone. Thickness of the vessels is constant throughout the scan as is their vascular signal. The vessels fan out and interconnect to form a complex pattern.

Interconnections between superficial and deep networks: The vascular network consists of

26 | Practical Handbook of OCT Angiography

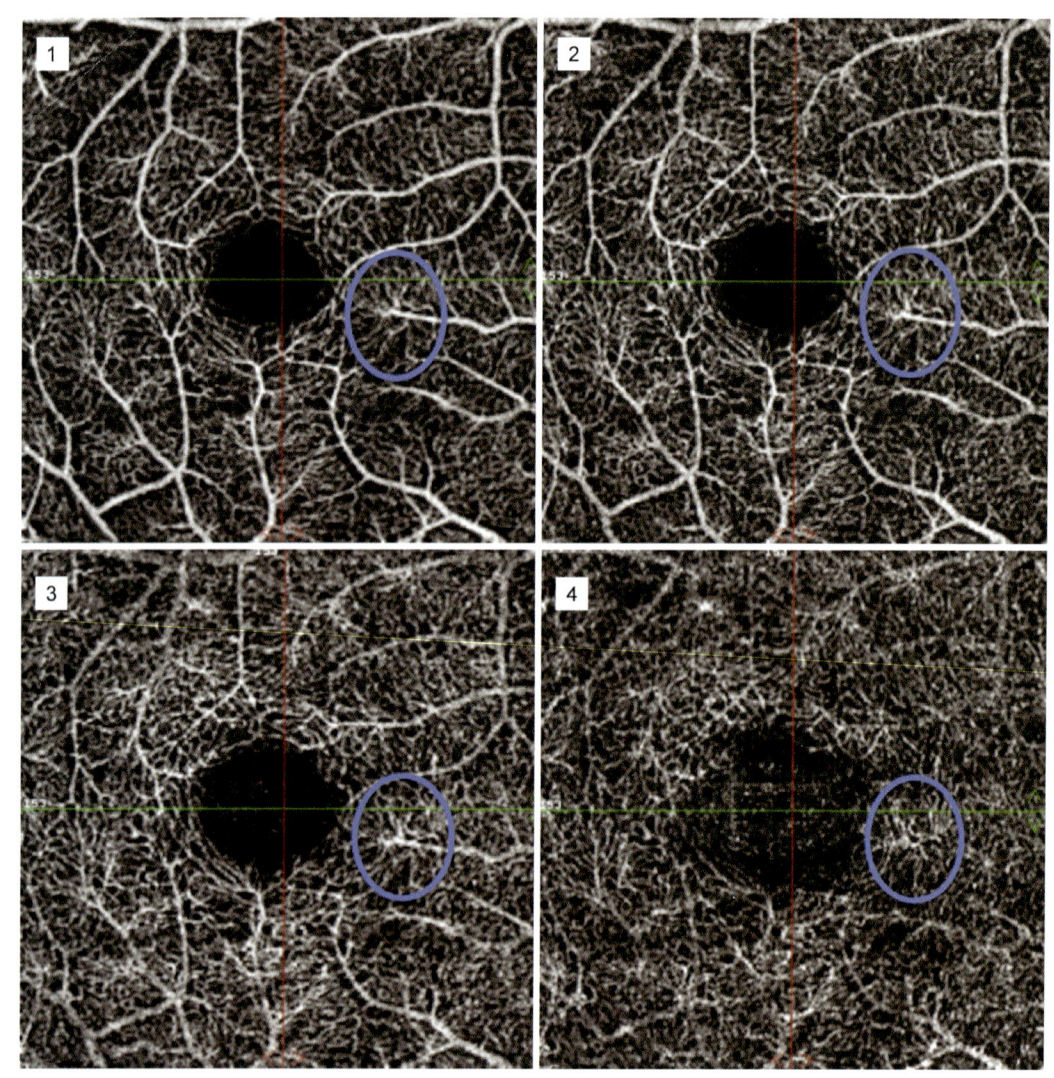

Figure 4.3 *Interconnections between superficial and deep networks:* Stack of consecutive *"en face"* OCT angiography scans (numbered from 1 to 4) from the superficial network to the deep network. The blue circle highlights different features of an interconnecting vascular branch, originating from the superficial net, going deeper and deeper, and eventually fanning out in the deep plexus

small vertical interconnecting anastomoses between the superficial and deeper vessels of the same deep plexus. The interconnecting vascular branches originate from the superficial net, go deeper and deeper, eventually fanning out in the deep plexus. From each lower extremity of the vertical anastomoses, horizontal vessels fan out and interconnect to form a complex pattern **(Fig. 4.3)**.

In fluorescein angiography, both plexuses overlap and therefore, they can neither be distinguished nor assessed separately. The contemporary visualization of both plexuses does not make it possible to analyze the superficial and deep vascular features that may be involved individually or separately in the various pathological processes. In healthy eyes, the superficial plexus consists of larger vessels with respect to the deep complex. Both plexuses are distributed according to a centripetal pattern around the avascular foveolar zone. The deep plexus consists of small fan shaped vessels that interconnect to form a complex pattern.

With fluorescein angiography, the vascular tree and therefore, the vessel morphology cannot be directly visualized; what is seen is the result of intravascular fluorescein. This effect is particularly evident in the case of retinal walls lesions and hence the dye leakage or pooling masks the real aspect of the vessels.

The OCT angiography precisely demonstrates the intravascular flow without the use of a dye. While this warrants a good visualization of the vessels, it does entail newer methods of imaging interpretation. There is a need for newer diagnostic parameters for vascular disorders.

One of the present limitations of OCT angiography is the size of the scan area involving the macular region alone (3 × 3 mm–6 × 6 mm). In the near future, a full field will be obtained and provide greater information and offer better detail. Another limitation is with respect to the currently available software for visualizing the structures under the retinal pigment epithelium (RPE).

BIBLIOGRAPHY

1. Carpineto P, Mastropasqua R, Marchini G, et al. Reproducibility and repeatability of foveal avascular zone measurements in healthy subjects by optical coherence tomography angiography. Br J Ophthalmol, 2015. [Epub ahead of print].
2. Druault A. Appareil de la Vision. Traité d'Anatomie Humaine. Poirier et Charpy, 1911;1: 1018.
3. Duke-Elder S. The Anatomy of Visual System. London, United Kingdom. 1961;2:372-6.
4. Hogan M, Alvarado J, Weddell JE. Histology of the Human Eye—An Atlas and Textbook. Philadelphia, PA: WB Saunders; 1971.
5. Huang D, Swanson EA, Lin CP, et al. Optical coherence tomography. Science. 1991;254: 1178-81.
6. Jia Y, Bailey ST, Wilson DJ, et al. Quantitative optical coherence tomography angiography of choroidal neovascularization in age-related macular degeneration. Ophthalmology. 2014; 121:1435-44.
7. Jia Y, Tan O, Tokayer J, et al. Split-spectrum amplitude decorrelation angiography with optical coherence tomography. Opt Express. 2012;20: 4710-25.
8. Redslob E. Anatomie du Globe Oculaire. Traité d'Ophtalmologie. Paris, France: Masson, édit, 1939;5:382.
9. Savastano MC, Lumbroso B, Rispoli M. In vivo characterization of retinal vascularization morphology using optical coherence tomography angiography. Retina. 2015;35:2196-203.
10. Spaide RF, Klancnik JM Jr, Cooney MJ. Retinal vascular layers imaged by fluorescein angiography and optical coherence tomography angiography. JAMA Ophthalmol. 2015;133:45-50.

5

Diabetic Retinopathy and Optical Coherence Tomography Angiography

Maria Cristina Savastano, Marco Rispoli, Bruno Lumbroso

INTRODUCTION

Diabetic retinopathy (DR) is one of the major ocular diabetic complications that can lead to blindness, as symptoms are not apparent till the later stages of the complication when lesions are already advanced, thereby limiting the efficacy of treatment.

The main risk factors associated with early onset and rapidly evolving retinopathy are the *duration* of diabetes, glycometabolic *imbalance*, poorly controlled *arterial hypertension*, and concomitant *dyslipidemia*. The most recent classification of DR was developed in 2001 by the American Academy of Ophthalmology (AAO) and approved in February, 2003.

Even though the universally accepted method for assessment of diabetes-related vascular anomalies is fluorescein angiography, there is increasing clinical use of optical coherence tomography (OCT) angiography. OCT angiography does not require the use of contrast dye and visualizes retinal circulation by using a dedicated software called the split-spectrum amplitude-decorrelation angiography (SSADA). OCT angiography with SSADA technology provides a detailed view of the vascular anomalies of the retina by a detailed, actual *stratigraphic* examination of its diverse layers. Often, OCT angiography highlights diabetes-induced lesions that are not obvious on ophthalmoscopy or structural OCT analysis (**Figs 5.1A to C**).

In diabetic patients, OCT angiography demonstrates some retinal alterations very clearly. Foveal avascular zone (FAZ) enlargement and microaneurysms are frequent findings. The provision of separately examining the superficial and deep retinal vascular plexus on OCT angiography makes it possible to delineate the retinal involvement in various diabetic lesions. For instance, *widening of the foveal avascular zone (FAZ)* is best seen in the superficial capillary plexus, while the sacciform dilatations of *microaneurysms* are best seen in the deep capillary plexus (**Figs 5.2A to C**).

Microaneurysms can be visualized on OCT angiography only in the presence of intravessel flow. Thus, thrombosed microaneurysms are silent and undetected on OCT angiography. In addition, microaneurysms with very slow flow are also silent and missed by the SSADA system.

The analysis of the widening of the FAZ corresponds to the study of ischemic maculopathy.

- The presence of *cystoid macular edema* in OCT angiography is recorded as absence of flow due to the "sliding" of retinal tissue linked to intraretinal cystic spaces. This visualization is more marked when analyzing the deep vascular plexus (**Figs 5.3A and B**). In the presence of macular edema, the OCT angiography analysis of both plexuses can recognize capillary distortion and vessel congestion. Vascular congestion is greatest at the edges of the ischemia.

With OCT angiography, the phenomenon of *capillary dropout* can also be appreciated. This phenomenon is less clear when analyzing the superficial vascular plexus and corresponds to the disappearance of the ramification of small capillaries in the ischemic areas (**Figs 5.4A and B**).

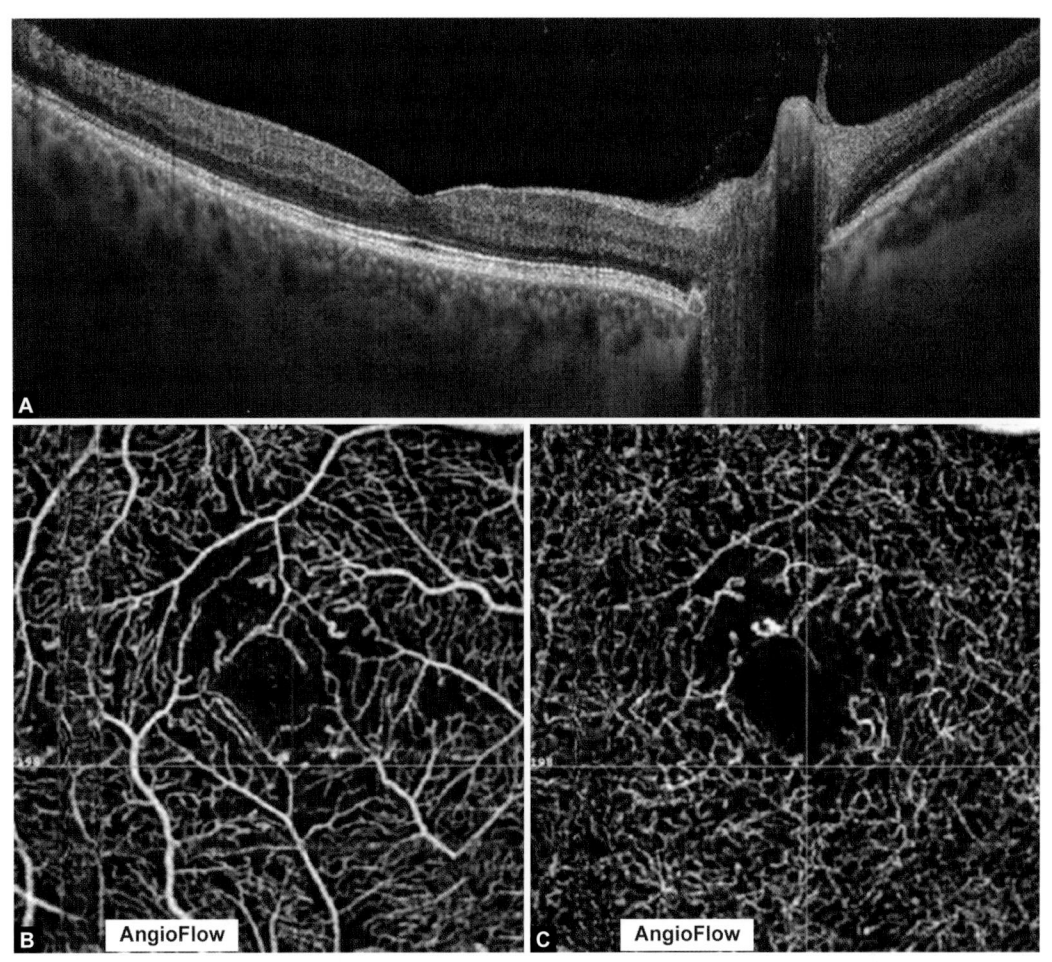

Figures 5.1A to C (A) Structural optical coherence tomography (OCT) of an eye with diabetic retinopathy where there is no major morphologic disruption except for a focal alteration of the juxtafoveal retinal profile; (B) OCT angiography of the superficial vascular plexus where an ischemic maculopathy with a widening of the foveal avascular zone (FAZ) and dilatation of the juxtafoveal vessels are seen; (C) OCT angiography of the deep vascular plexus shows vascular congestion microaneurysms and texture rarefaction

30 Practical Handbook of OCT Angiography

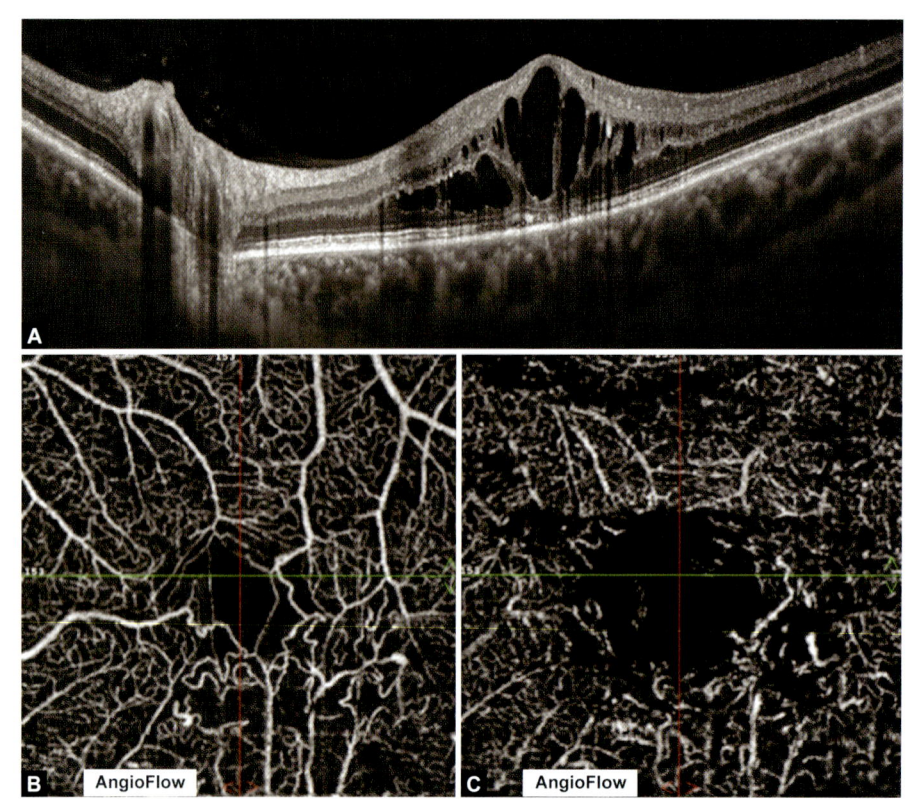

Figures 5.2A to C (A) B-scan structural OCT of an eye with diabetic retinopathy and cystoid macular edema; (B) OCT angiography demonstrates widening of the FAZ at the superficial plexus and many vessel convolutions; (C) OCT angiography at the deep plexus is partially altered by the intraretinal cystic spaces but shows a diffused vascular alteration with vascular congestion

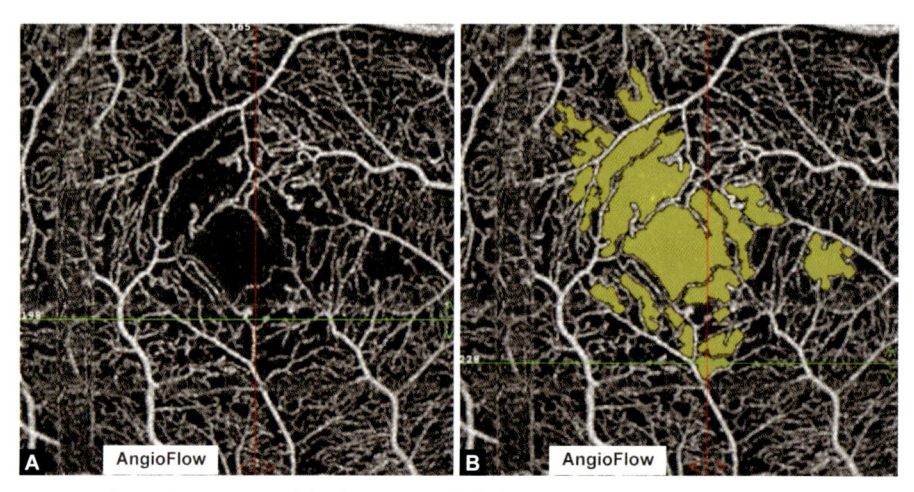

Figures 5.3A and B OCT angiography of an eye with diabetic retinopathy and ischemic maculopathy: (A) The areas of low perfusion around the FAZ (dropout) corresponding to the superficial vascular plexus can be recognized; (B) The same areas are highlighted by the calculation integrated software "no flow"

Diabetic Retinopathy and Optical Coherence Tomography Angiography | **31**

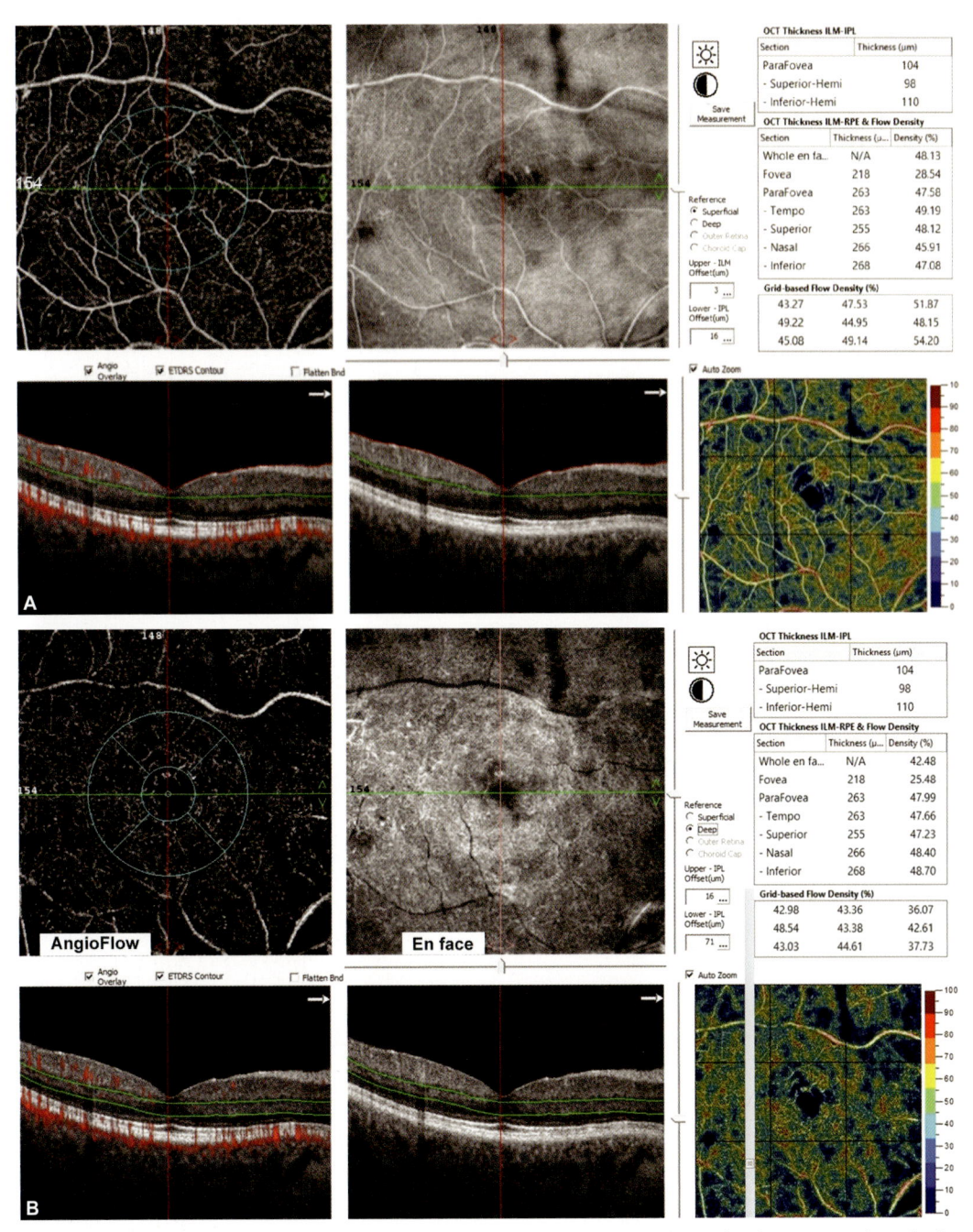

Figures 5.4A and B OCT angiography of an eye with diabetic retinopathy and ischemic maculopathy by using flow density analysis: (A) Flow density at the superficial plexus; (B) Flow density in the deep capillary plexus

OBJECTIVE QUANTITATIVE ANALYSIS

Flow area: With the evolution of the OCT Angiography software it is possible to show the area involved in the widening of the FAZ and the ischemic areas (dropout) **(Fig. 5.4A)**.

Flow density: The integration of this new algorithm enables objective estimation of flow density in any layer **(Fig. 5.4B)**.

BIBLIOGRAPHY

1. Agemy SA, Scripsema NK, Shah CM, et al. Retinal vascular perfusion density mapping using optical coherence tomography angiography in normals and diabetic retinopathy patients. Retina. 2015; 35(11):2353-63.
2. Hwang TS, Jia Y, Gao SS, et al. Optical coherence tomography angiography features of diabetic retinopathy. Retina. 2015;35(11):2371-6.
3. Ishibazawa A, Nagaoka T, Takahashi A, et al. Optical Coherence Tomography Angiography in Diabetic Retinopathy: A Prospective Pilot Study. Am J Ophthalmol. 2015;160(1):35-44.

6

Vascular Occlusions

Marco Rispoli, Bruno Lumbroso, Maria Cristina Savastano, Jean Francois Le Rouic, Pascal Peronnet

BRANCH OR CENTRAL VEIN OCCLUSIONS

Marco Rispoli, Bruno Lumbroso, Maria Cristina Savastano

CENTRAL RETINAL VEIN OCCLUSION AND VENOUS BRANCH OCCLUSION

Retinal venous occlusions are acute vascular events that may affect the central retinal vein, one of its branches or a portion of a small branch. Fluorescein angiography has made it possible to highlight vessel anomalies associated with occlusions. In recent years, since the introduction of optical coherence tomography (OCT) angiography it is further possible to separately study the occluded areas in the retinal layers.

Differences between Fluorescein Angiography and OCT Angiography

In eyes affected by venous branch occlusions, OCT angiography highlights the two vascular networks comprising the capillary dropout areas corresponding to the capillary dropout areas seen on fluorescein angiography (FAG) **(Figs 6.1A and B)**. These areas are also seen more sharply because there is no masking effect caused by leakage of dye as seen in FAG intermediate and later images. These areas of occlusion are evident both at the superficial and deeper vascular plexus levels, even though the no-flow areas are more evident when analyzing the superficial plexus.

In the deep vascular plexus, vascular congestion is more obvious with evidence of an uneven coexistence of capillaries, some with increased caliber and others with a smaller caliber or occluded. Thus, a coarse net is visible where some meshes are larger and sparser with a fine, grayish texture **(Fig. 6.2)**.

With OCT angiography, the vascular network can therefore, be seen more sharply with clear demonstration of the arterial-venous anastomoses and the vascular loops **(Fig. 6.3)**. This features are not visible with fluorescein angiography owing to dye leakage affecting the FAG intermediate and late slides.

The ischemic or low flow districts are seen as areas where the capillaries are sparse and more obvious against a gray background. The texture, which can vary from fine to coarse, needs to be studied and noted. Often, inside the capillary dropout areas, capillaries appear truncated, with sharp sections. Sometimes arterial-venous anastomoses with capillary layers of the deep vascular network are seen at the level of the inner nuclear layer.

Retinal edema zones are not easily appreciated on OCT angiography as there is no dye staining. However, at times a widening and distortion of the capillary network meshes can be noticed, and this indirect data is used by OCT angiography

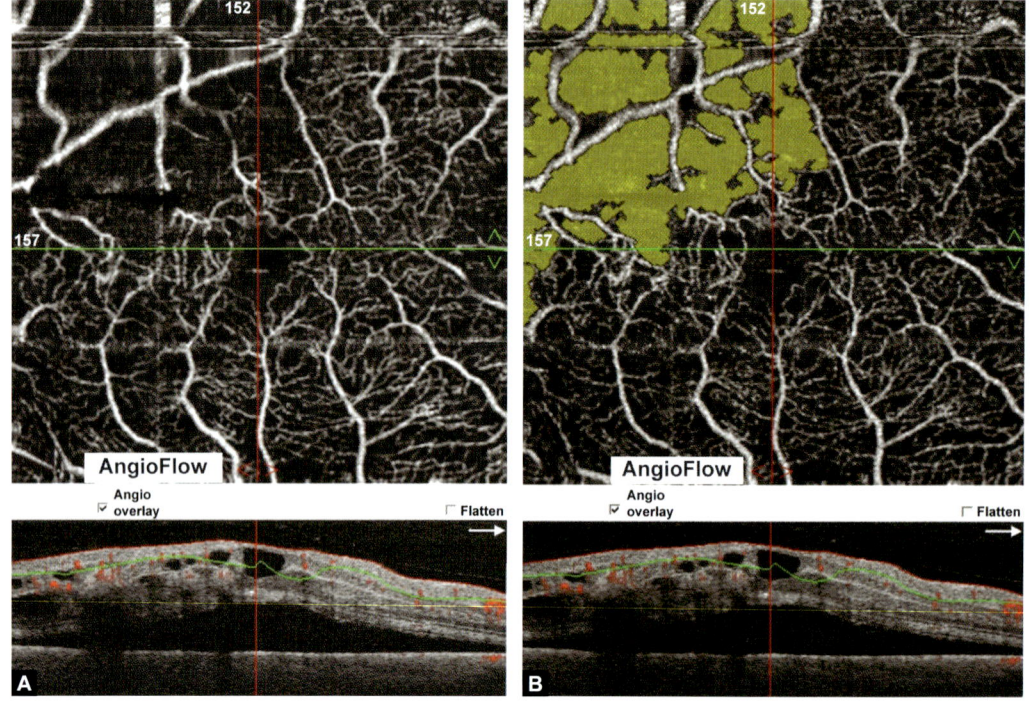

Figures 6.1A and B *Capillary drop out in both networks.* OCT angiography highlights the two vascular networks with capillary dropout areas. Areas of occlusion are evident both at the superficial and deeper vascular plexus levels, however the no-flow areas are more evident when analyzing the superficial plexus. No flow areas are highlighted in yellow by the software

is analyzing edema. An advantage of the split-spectrum amplitude-decorrelation angiography (SSADA) algorithm, which allows almost total exclusion of structural data, is the ability to observe dark intraretinal edema cells associated with fine septa having low density where at times small vessels can be evidenced **(Fig. 6.4)**.

While fluorescein angiography shows vessel walls and its contents by dye staining, OCT angiography shows a very thin vessel that corresponds only to the lumen itself, surrounded by a dark area representing the thickened vessel wall. Thus, there is a sharp difference in the imaging results of fluorescein angiography and OCT angiography **(Figs 6.5 and 6.6)**.

Retinal hemorrhages are visible as masked areas but are less obvious with OCT angiography than with fluorescein angiography. In the ischemic areas, the background texture may vary from a pale gray to a grayish granulation.

OPTICAL COHERENCE TOMOGRAPHY ANGIOGRAPHY

Superficial Vascular Plexus

Changes in the structure of the superficial plexus can be observed in the presence of occlusions, mainly in case of macular ischemia. The areas of occlusion are evident not only in the study of the superficial vascular plexus but also on examining the deep plexus. The demarcations of no-flow areas, however, are more obvious when examining the superficial plexus. The arterial-venous anastomoses and the vascular loops are easily appreciated. In these cases, the vessel course is no longer linear but presents focal deviations; the wall thickness is irregular and discontinuous with focal segmentation and luminal narrowing; the course of the vessels has frequent abrupt interruptions with terminal dilatations around the avascular

Vascular Occlusions | 35

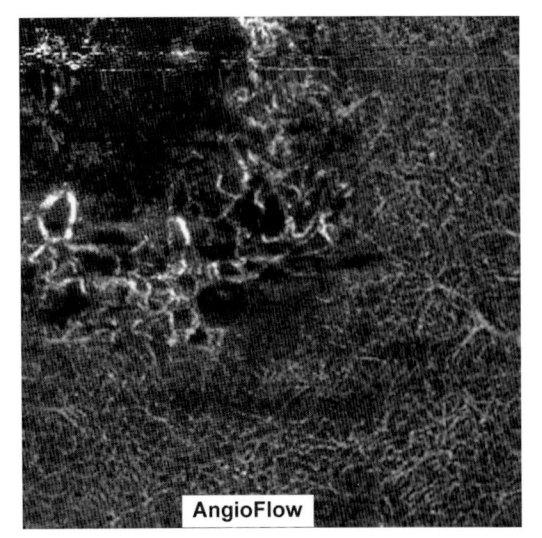

Figure 6.2 *Deep vascular plexus vascular congestion.* Vascular congestion is more obvious with evidence of an uneven coexistence of capillaries, some with increased caliber and others with a smaller caliber or occluded. A coarse vascular net is visible where some meshes are larger and sparser

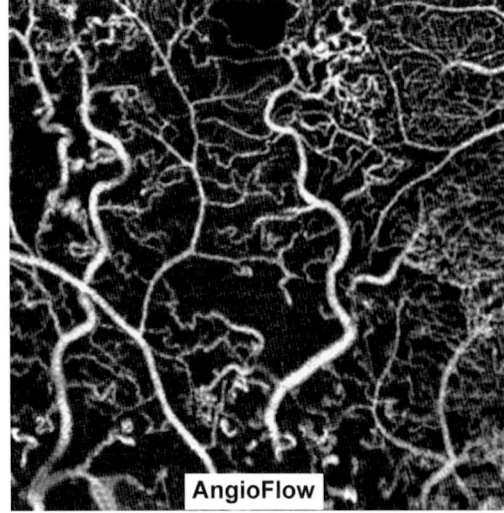

Figure 6.3 *Superficial vascular network.* Superficial vascular network is seen sharper with clear demonstration of the arterial-venous anastomoses and the vascular loops. These features are not visible with fluorescein angiography owing to dye leakage. Inside the dropout areas, capillaries appear truncated, with sharp sections. Some arterial-venous anastomoses with the deep vascular network are seen at the level of the inner nuclear layer

foveal zone. The foveal zone appears wider than in healthy individuals. The other findings observed, are the presence of many microvascular anomalies, increased vascular congestion of the deep plexus, and segmented vessel flow.

The no-flow areas and capillary dropout zones appear as districts where capillaries are sparse and more obvious.

In OCT angiography, the areas of retinal edema can be identified owing to an absence of dye leakage and is recognized by the presence of widening and distortion of the capillary network meshes and blurring of the widened capillaries.

Deep Vascular Plexus

The deep plexus shows major changes with venous occlusion, mainly in the ischemic areas. The capillary distribution is irregular with variations in vessel direction in the no-flow area. Dilated capillaries with increased caliber alternate with capillaries with reduced caliber or capillaries that are apparently closed. A coarse vascular net is visible with some meshes that are larger, sparser and have a fine grayish texture.

The vessels walls are thicker in the pathologic areas; vessels present multiple irregular shunts at various levels of the retina. The texture appears to be different in the affected vascular zone. An increase in vascular congestion is evident in the deep plexus. In addition, there are irregularities in vessel size, presence of localized dilatations, as well as aneurysms and microaneurysms of different sizes. Vascular congestion is mainly visible at the border between normal retina and the occluded zone.

Border Area between Normal and Occluded Area

Major alterations are demonstrated at the border between normal retina and the occluded area.

36 | Practical Handbook of OCT Angiography

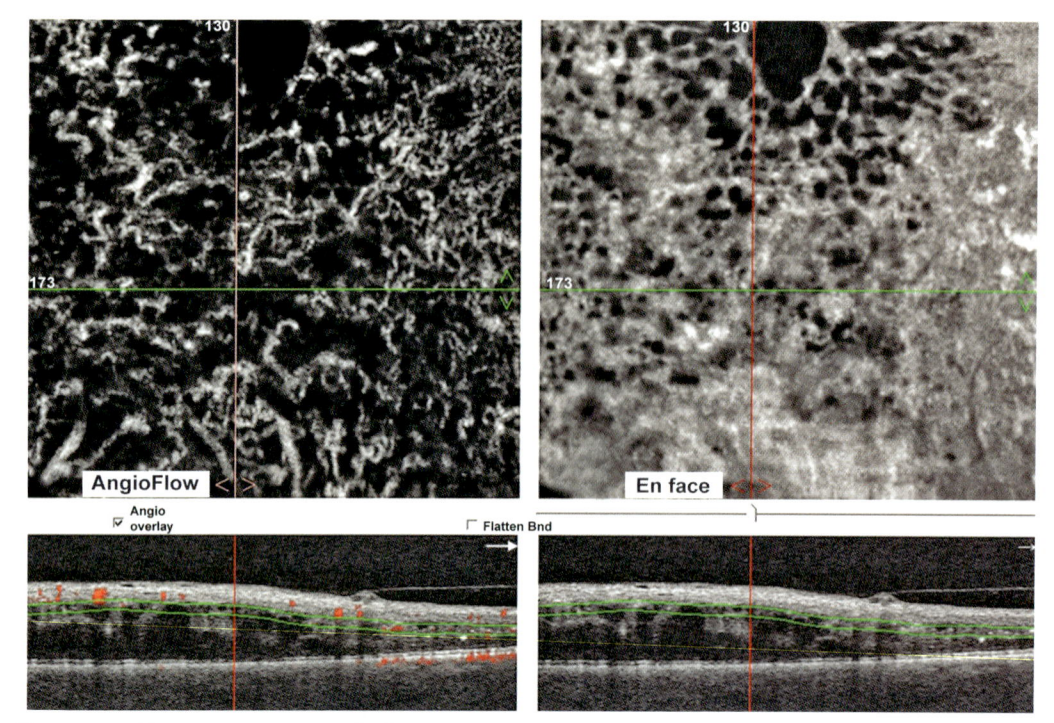

Figure 6.4 *Edematous areas.* Retinal edema zones are not easily appreciated on OCT angiography as there is no dye staining. At times a widening and distortion of the capillary network meshes can be noticed, and this indirect data is used by OCT angiography is analyzing edema. Dark intraretinal edema cells are associated with fine septa having low density

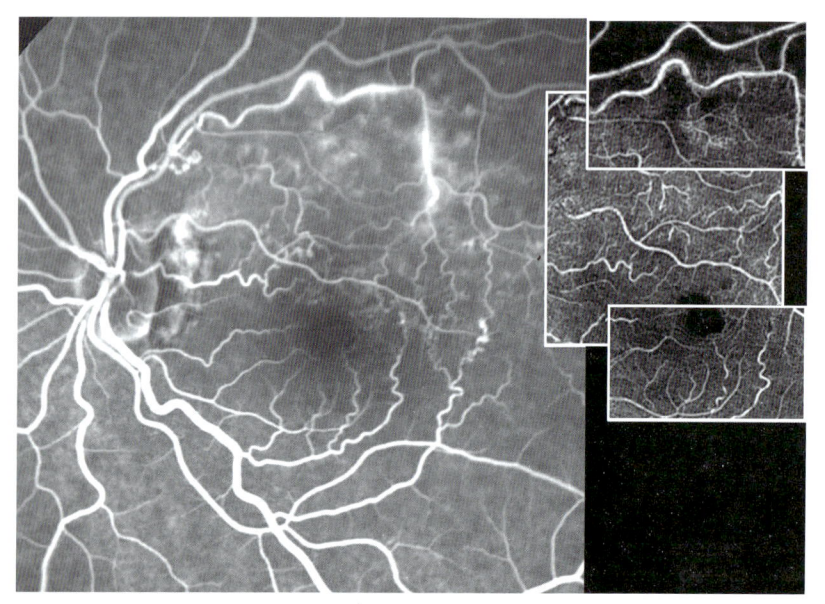

Figure 6.5 Branch retinal vein occlusion (BRVO) as seen with fluorescein angiography and OCT angiography. Note that there is no dye leakage in OCT angiography

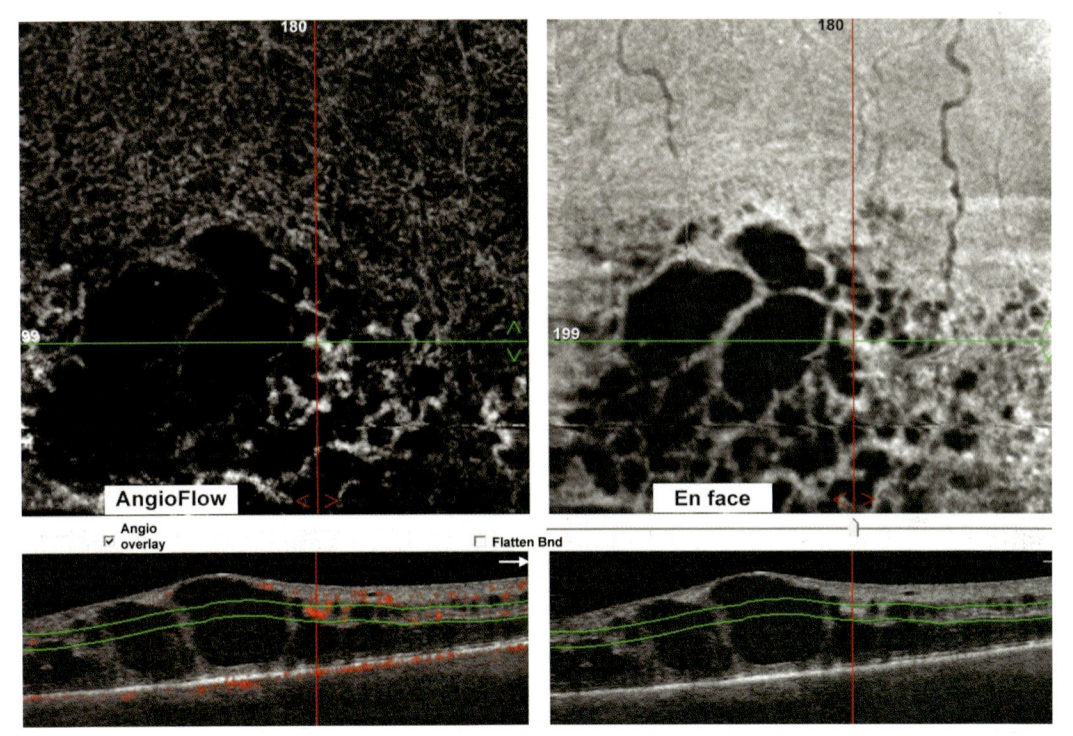

Figure 6.6 *Edematous areas*. Retinal edema areas show a widening and distortion of the capillary network meshes. Dark intraretinal edema cells are separated by fine low density septa

Some capillaries are dilated to varying degrees, while others are constricted or closed. The vascular net shows some larger meshes and some, which are smaller and sparser. The vessels consist of multiple irregular shunts in the various layers of the retina, more evident at the border between the normal and occluded retina. The texture is different in the no-flow area where the vascularization is affected. There is an increase in vascular congestion in the deep plexus where anomalies in vessel size, presence of localized dilatations, and aneurysms and microaneurysms of different sizes. Vascular congestion is also mainly observed at the margin between normal retina and no-flow area.

Avascular Foveal Zone

The avascular foveal zone is wider and less regular than in healthy individuals; the ischemic areas merge with the avascular zone thus widening the no-flow areas.

Central Retinal Vein Occlusion

In the acute phase of the occlusion process, hemorrhages and vascular congestion in the posterior pole decrease visibility of potential no-flow areas particularly if the resulting edema is significant. Vascular congestion affects both plexuses but the changes in the deep plexus are more marked and thus clearly evident **(Figs 6.7A and B)**.

Recent Retinal Ischemia

The OCT angiography makes it possible to highlight the main superficial vessels of the retina that are typically associated with loss of collateral branches following an ischemic event. In cases of recent ischemia this capillary dropout involves the superficial vascular plexus almost exclusively, while the morphology, caliber and reflectivity of the deep plexus capillaries is fairly preserved **(Fig. 6.8)**.

7

Type 1, Type 2 and Type 4 (Mixed) Choroidal Neovascularization

Bruno Lumbroso, Marco Rispoli

INTRODUCTION

Noninvasive optical coherence tomography (OCT) angiography allows for the study and classification of new vessels **(Table 7.1)**, highlighting their morphology, flow, and exact localization. Absence of dye staining, leakage and pooling are the factors that facilitate easy interpretation of OCT angiograms. The new vessels are highlighted with greater accuracy and allow for both qualitative and quantitative assessment. With OCT angiography, the intraretinal flows can be observed at each level. In the first modern classification of new vessels made 20 years ago, Gass differentiated visible vessels, or classical new vessels, which had a network that could clearly be seen on fluorescein angiography, from occult new vessels where fluorescein angiography could only demonstrate a slow and progressive dye leakage or oozing. More recently, Jung and Freund have developed a new classification that has been widely adopted.

In age-related macular degeneration, the exudative form shows anomalous new vessels growing from the choroid and choriocapillaris. They may develop either between the Bruch's membrane and the pigmented epithelium, in which case they are Type 1 subepithelial new vessels (referred to as occult new vessels until recently), or they may develop in the pre-epithelial subretinal space, in which case they are Type 2 new vessels (previously referred to as classical new vessels).

Exudate and hemorrhages can be seen in both types of new vessels.

In Type 1, the exudate has fibrous and vascular content and results in flat detachment of pigment epithelium.

In Type 2, subretinal fluid and cystoid edema are almost always present. Hemorrhages and alterations of the outer retinal layers can be observed along with severe lesions in the photoreceptor layer.

Type 3 is dealt with in the next chapter.

In Type 4, or mixed type, both Type 1 and Type 2 new vessels are seen in the same lesion, with a flat detachment of pigment epithelium, subretinal fluid, cystoid edema as well as hemorrhages and alterations in the outer retinal layers.

OCT angiography represents a step forward in diagnostic imaging, and is a fast, precise and clear way of highlighting the choroidal retinal vascularization without the difficulties caused by dye leakage or pooling. The split-spectrum amplitude decorrelation angiography (SSADA) technology developed by David Huang and Yali Jia, is currently the most commonly used algorithm in OCT angiographic studies worldwide.

Table 7.1 Classification of new vessels

Jung and Freund, AJO 2014

- *Type 1*: Underneath the pigmented epithelium (40%)
- *Type 2*: Subretinal (9%)
- *Type 3*: Intraretinal (24%)
- *Type 4*: Mixed (17%)

Other types

- Myopic
- CRSC CNV
- Residual new vessels in fibrous scars

Abbreviations: CRSC, central serous chorioretinopathy; CNV, choroidal neovascularization

While imaging with fluorescein angiography and indocyanine green angiography overlay all the retinal structures in two-dimensional flat images, OCT angiography enables the study of new vessels separately at different levels of the retina and choroid, facilitating the assessment of choroidal neovascularization (CNV), layer by layer, as well as globally. Since OCT angiography does not entail the injection of any contrast substance, the images are not affected by dye leakage, staining or pooling and allow accurate study of the branching and ramification of abnormal vessels.

ASSESSING NEW VESSELS

Choroidal new vessels are assessed and classified on the basis of their morphology, the types of subdivisions of their branches, the presence or absence of loops, and their capillary density. Some peripheral loops may merge at the extremities of radial vessels, while other forms of CNV may have the appearance of a bare tree **(Table 7.2)**.

The new vessels are therefore, subdivided according to the following characteristics:

Morphology

New vessels are described as having the appearance of a Medusa head (referring to the mythological monster Medusa), coral, bicycle-wheel, fan or sea-fan, dead tree, or tangled network of threads and vascular loops **(Table 7.3)**.

Density

Capillaries may be densely packed, thin and numerous, or, as a result of the arterialization following repeated recurrences, they may be thicker, straighter, rigid and lack thinner capillaries.

Loops

The loops are mainly located i_ where they can merge, and ha _ppearances described as wheel-shaped CNV, fans or corals. They may be frequent, rare and thin or dense within the arborizations. Loops are rarely found in tangled new vessels or in bare tree CNV.

A recently developed Optovue software allows quantification of the flow surface in neovascular membranes. The software highlights the flow surface in yellow, enabling interpretation without any further difficult and time-consuming maneuvers. Since OCT angiography can be frequently repeated, it is easier to follow-up both treated and untreated new vessels.

TYPE 1 NEW VESSELS

Type 1 new vessels (formerly called occult) develop under the pigment epithelium and result in its flat elevation. The neovascularization often occurs between the elevated pigment epithelium and Bruch's membrane **(Table 7.4)**.

Clinical Features

Type 1 new vessels appear under the retinal pigment epithelium (RPE), often between the

Table 7.2 CNV features
• Morphology
• Capillary density
• Branches subdivision and arborization
• Loops present or lacking
• Vessels thin or thick
• Straight or sinuous

Table 7.3 Morphology
• Coral shaped
• Fan shaped
• Medusa head
• Wheel shaped
• Tangled
• Bare tree shaped
• Filamentary
• Star shaped
• Tuft shaped
• Glomerular

Table 7.4 Morphology of type 1 CNV
• Coral shaped
• Fan shaped
• Medusa head
• Wheel shaped
• Tangled arborization
• Bare tree shaped
• Filamentary

Abbreviation: CNV, choroidal neovascularization

elevated pigment epithelium and the Bruch's membrane. The elevated RPE may look stratified if there is fibrovascular tissue proliferation. Fluid is seen under the detached RPE and is often associated with subretinal fluid. The risk of tear of the elevated pigment epithelium is high. Without treatment, Type 1 CNV will evolve towards a fibrovascular plaque. Hemorrhages and outer retinal layer lesions are frequent as the condition evolves to its later phases. Alterations of the outer retina with severe lesions involving the ellipsoid and photoreceptors are consistently observed. Fibrosis sets in at a later stage.

Fluorescein Angiography Features

Early leakage hyperfluorescence is seen, which increases slowly with progressive oozing of the dye. The lesion margins are blurred, and the fluid leakage is irregular. CNV is seen as a blurred hyperfluorescent area.

Indocyanine Green Features

In the very early frames, the feeder vessel and its ramifications can be appreciated. In late indocyanine green (ICG) frames, a plaque with sharp margins can be observed. More rarely, the margins are blurred or there are two or three overlapping plaques. Occasionally, hyperfluorescent dots may be seen.

Structural OCT Features

Very frequently, a flat irregular or undulated pigment epithelium elevation may be noted. Between the pigment epithelium elevation and Bruch's membrane, fluid or fibrovascular tissue are present. Around the lesion, alterations, irregularities, and thickening of the ellipsoid zone are seen. The neuroepithelium is partially disrupted. Structural OCT shows fibrous layers under the elevated epithelium. There is the danger that the elevated pigment epithelium may tear.

OCT Angiography Features

Type 1 vessels always appear under the pigment epithelium initially and no flow is observed in the nonvascularized zone. The new vessels may later spread out into the avascular area of the external retina. The neovascular network is often extensive and has high flows.

Morphology is varied and the branches have different appearances. There are new vessels with shapes described as medusa-head, coral, bicycle-wheel, fan, dead tree, tangled network, filaments and vascular loops. The observed morphology leaves no room for uncertainty about diagnosis because features are so different from normal vascularization.

The capillaries may be dense or sparse, the vessels may be thin and numerous, or, as a result of arterialization following repeated relapses, they may be thicker, straighter, and rigid with loss of thinner capillaries.

The loops are mostly seen in the periphery of the CNV and contribute to the formation of wheel, fan, medusa-head or coral-shaped new vessels. They may be frequent, rare and thin, or dense with complex arborization. Loops are rare in filament-like tangled new vessels and in bare-tree-like new vessels.

The vascular complex almost always has a feeder trunk or a bundle of feeder vessels. Type 1 new vessels have been defined as "mature" by Sarraf and Waheed. They present branches that radiate into all directions, in the shape of a medusa-head, coral, bicycle-wheel or sea-fan on only one side.

The *filament-like new vessels*, simple or tangled, are occasionally observed in age-related macular degeneration, though they are more typically seen in chronic epitheliopathy (in 20–30 % of cases).

The loops are mainly seen in the CNV periphery, where they form the bicycle-wheel, fan and coral-like new vessels. They may be frequently seen, and appear rare and thin, or densely packed within the arborizations.

Type 1 new vessels generally have a larger surface than Type 2 new vessels (**Figs 7.1 to 7.7**).

Perilesional Dark Halo

As demonstrated by David Huang, Yali Jia and David Bailey, there is always a halo or dark circle around the new vessels. In their opinion this could be attributed to morphological changes or blood flow alterations in the choriocapillaris, or due to screen effect.

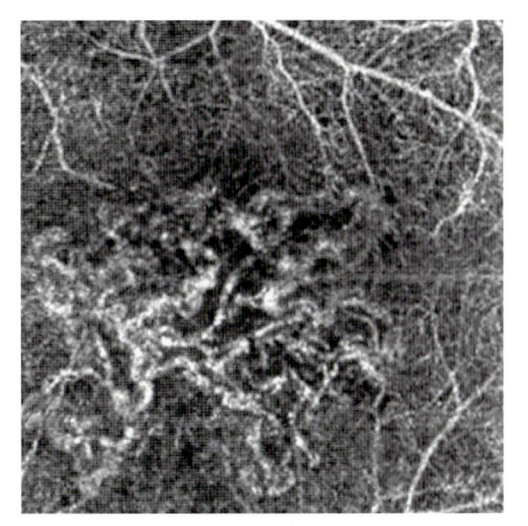

Type 1, Type 2 and Type 4 (Mixed) Choroidal Neovascularization | **47**

Figure 7.1 OCT angiography. Type 1 new vessels with varied morphology. The new vessels have the shape of a medusa-head

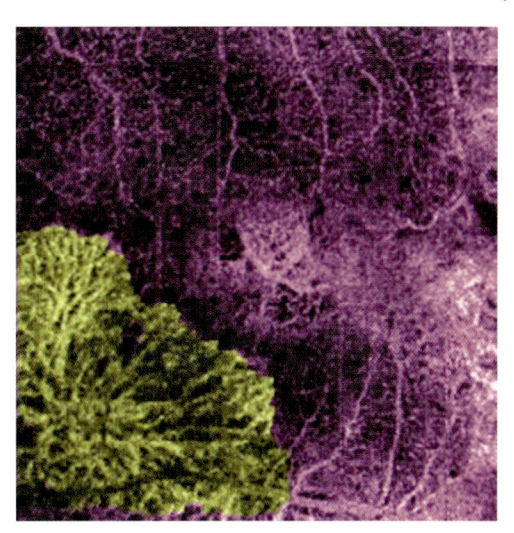

Figure 7.2 OCT angiography. Type 1 new vessels: The new vessels have the shape of coral. The vascular loops are mainly seen in the periphery

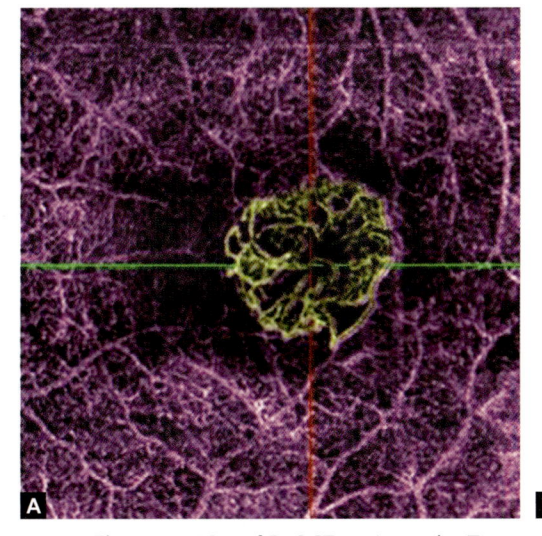

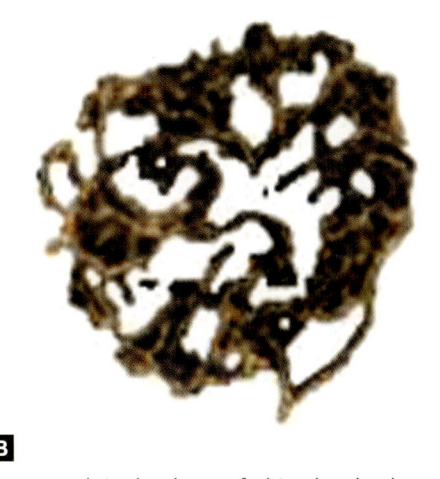

Figures 7.3A and B OCT angiography. Type 1 new vessels in the shape of a bicycle-wheel. The loops are mainly in the periphery

TYPE 2 NEW VESSELS

These vessels, previously referred to as "classical new vessels", develop in the subretinal space (pre-epithelium new vessels), above the pigmented epithelium. They may penetrate into the outer avascular retinal area. Their size is, in general, smaller than Type 1 new vessels **(Figs 7.8 to 7.10 and Table 7.5)**.

Clinical Features of Type 2 New Vessels

Intraretinal fluid (diffuse edema and cystoid edema) is always observed along with fluid pooling

48 | Practical Handbook of OCT Angiography

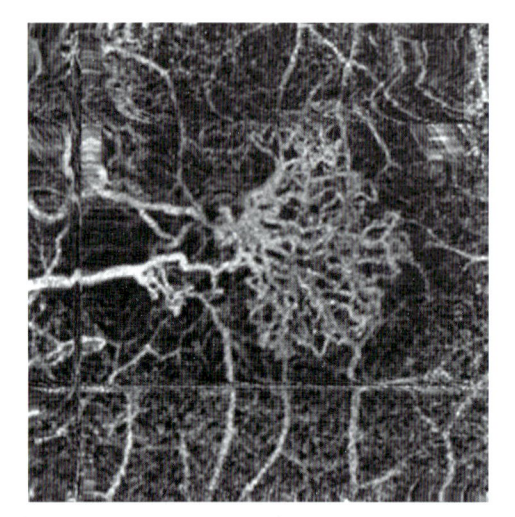

Figure 7.4 OCT angiography. Type 1 new vessels in the shape of a fan. The vascular loops are mainly seen in the periphery

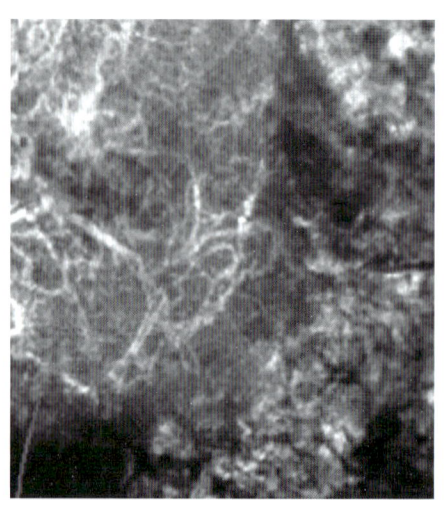

Figure 7.5 OCT angiography. Type 1 new vessels in the shape of a bare tree. Loops are rarely found in new vessels that look like a bare tree

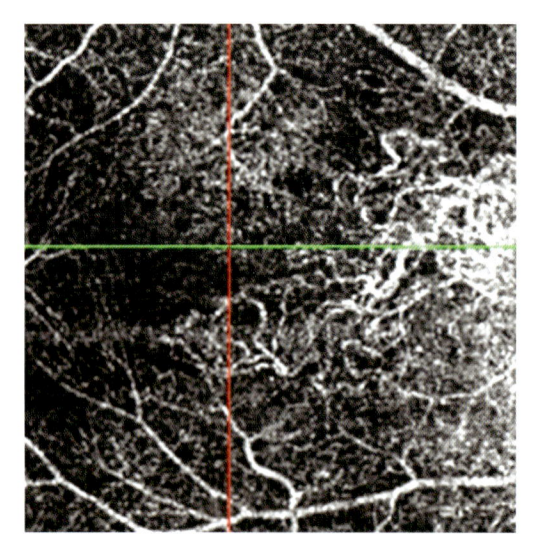

Figure 7.6 OCT angiography. Type 1 new vessels forming a tangled network

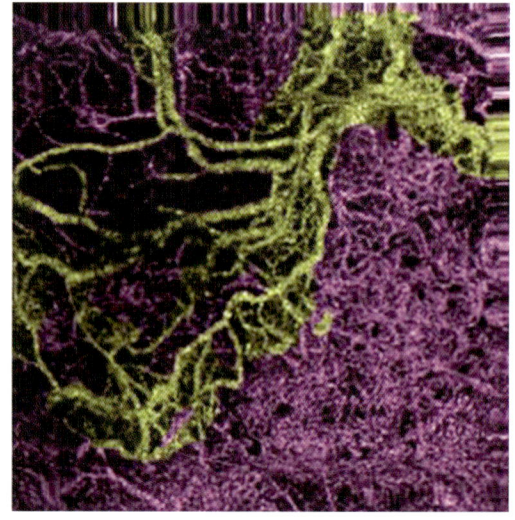

Figure 7.7 OCT angiography. Type 1 filamentary or tangled new vessels are occasionally observed in age-related macular degeneration, though they are more common in case of epitheliopathy. Loops are rarely seen

underneath the retina, with occasional flat retinal detachment. Pigment epithelium detachments are generally not observed, while hemorrhages are frequent. In the absence of treatment, the new vessels grow rapidly, at rates of about 9 mm a day.

Fluorescein Angiography Features

Type 2 classical new vessels are smaller than Type 1 occult new vessels. Hemorrhages are

Type 1, Type 2 and Type 4 (Mixed) Choroidal Neovascularization | 49

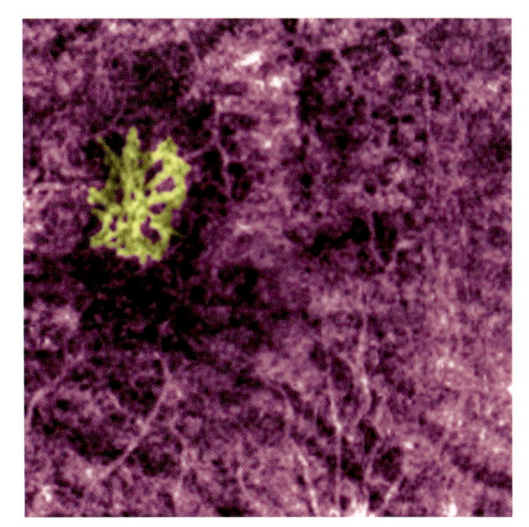

Figure 7.8 OCT angiography. Type 2 new vessels: Type 2 new vessels generally have smaller surface area than Type 1 new vessels. The new vessels have the appearance of a bicycle-wheel. Vascular loops are mainly seen in the periphery

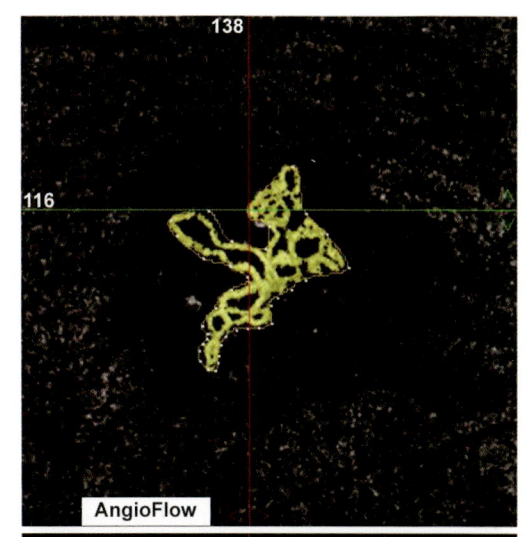

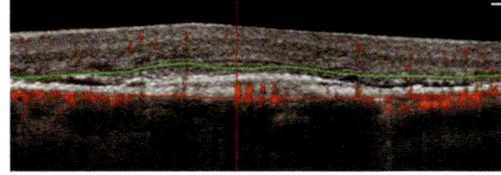

Figure 7.10 OCT angiography. Type 2 arterialized new vessels: After repeated treatment, arterialization occurs wherein the capillaries become wider, thicker and straighter, and often look rigid. The thinner capillaries disappear

Table 7.5 Morphology of type 2 CNV
• Coral shaped
• Fan shaped
• Medusa head
• Wheel shaped
• Rounded
• Arborization
• Star shaped

Abbreviation: CNV, choroidal neovascularization

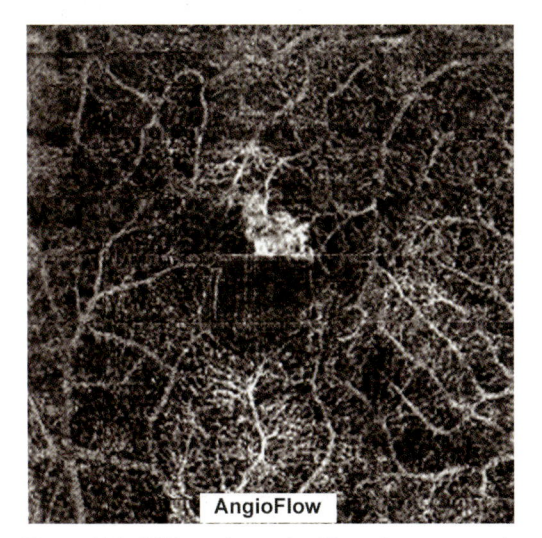

Figure 7.9 OCT angiography. Type 2 new vessels: Type 2 new vessels generally have smaller surface area than Type 1 new vessels. The new vessels have the appearance of a fan-like shape

frequent. Hyperfluorescence is more marked, and has sharper margins than in Type 1 new vessels. Occasionally, the new vessels show a bicycle-wheel shape with central feeder vessels and merging loops at the periphery of the lesions. New vessels grow rapidly, about 9 mm a day, and amounting to 50–60 mm in one week.

Structural OCT Features

Retinal thickness increases and constantly involves the neuroepithelium. There are small cells of cystoid and diffuse edema. The hyperreflective small speckles described by Coscas are almost always present along with hemorrhages. Occasionally, there are intraretinal hyperreflective areas with margins that are not too sharp.

OCT Angiography Features

Initially, Type 2 new vessels are always located above the pigmented epithelium. Flow is always seen in the avascular area. The new vessels subsequently spread more deeply into the outer retinal avascular area. The area of the neovascular network is smaller than in Type 1 new vessels. The flow is usually high and the morphology is varied though not to the extent seen in Type 1. The most frequent morphology found are the bicycle-wheel and fan-like shapes. The morphology of the new vessels is clearly different from normal vascularization.

In terms of density, the capillaries are often packed and the vessels are thin and numerous. Repeated treatment results in the phenomenon of *arterialization*: the capillaries become wider, thicker and straighter with a rigid appearance, while the thinner capillaries disappear. The loops are mostly in the periphery and they contribute to the appearance of wheel and fan-like new vessels. These may be frequent and thin, or rare and dense when they are located within the arborization.

The neovascular membrane always presents a large feeder trunk or a bundle of feeder vessels with centrifugal branches in the shape of a bicycle-wheel or a sea-fan on only one side. Type 2 new vessels, also called classical new vessels, generally have a smaller surface area than Type 1 occult vessels.

Fluid is present, especially when the new vessels penetrate into the neuroepithelium: pooling of subretinal fluid and small cells of cystoid edema. Hemorrhages and alterations in the external retinal layers are also seen with fibrosis and severe lesions involving the photoreceptors.

There is always a halo or dark halo around the new vessels secondary to morphological changes, screen effect or alterations in the blood flow of the choriocapillaris.

TYPE 3 NEW VESSELS

These are dealt with in another chapter by Souied et al. (**Table 7.6**).

TYPE 4 NEW VESSELS (MIXED TYPE)

For the first time in imaging, OCT angiography has enabled an accurate study of these complex membranes that spread beyond a single retinal layer. OCT angiography provides the ability to separately highlight these membranes and visualize them in different colors ensuring greater accuracy in their diagnosis (**Table 7.7**).

This type of CNV includes two or more parallel, flat, stratified vascular formations overlaid at several levels. Type 2 new vessels above the pigment epithelium have a rounded or fan-like shape, with loops at the periphery. Deeper down, underneath the pigment epithelium but above Bruch's membrane, one or more larger

Table 7.6 Morphology of type 3 CNV

- Tuft shaped
- Star shaped

Abbreviation: CNV, choroidal neovascularization

Table 7.7 Morphology of type 4 CNV

Type 4 CNV include two or more vascular parallel flat stratified formations overlaid at several levels: Type 2 new vessels above the pigment epithelium. Deeper down, underneath the pigment epithelium but above Bruch's membrane, one or more larger and irregular Type 1 CNV

Morphology of type 1 CNV

- Coral shaped
- Fan shaped
- Medusa head
- Wheel shaped
- Tangled
- Arborization
- Bare tree
- Filamentary

Morphology of type 2 CNV

- Coral shaped
- Fan shaped
- Medusa head
- Wheel shaped
- Rounded
- Arborization
- Star shaped

Abbreviation: CNV, choroidal neovascularization

and irregular Type 1 neovascular membranes are present.

Clinical Features

They form in two or more layers, above the pigment epithelium and also between the flat wavy elevation of the pigment epithelium and the Bruch's membrane. The elevation contents often appear stratified. There is fluid under the detached epithelium along with subretinal fluid. If untreated, this gradually evolves into a fibrovascular plaque. There are hemorrhages, edema and hard exudates, disruption of outer retinal layers, and severe lesions involving the photoreceptors. Fibrosis appears at a later stage.

Fluorescein Angiography Features

The early, diffuse hyperfluorescence increases slowly and progressively. The margins are blurred and the leakage is irregular, caused due to oozing of the dye. These findings are due to Type 1 occult new vessels. There are also other aspects associated with Type 2 classical new vessels. Hemorrhages are frequent. Hyperfluorescence is more marked than in Type 1 new vessels and has sharper margins, wheel-shaped appearance, along with a central feeder vessel and peripheral merging loops. Therefore, in early frames, diffuse gradually increasing hyperfluorescence coexists with areas of marked hyperfluorescence with sharper margins.

ICG Features

In the early frames, the feeder vessel can be seen along with its ramifications. In the later stages, a plaque is observed, which generally has sharp margins. Rarely, the margins are blurred with occasional overlapping plaques.

Structural OCT Features

New vessels are observed between the flat elevation of the pigmented epithelium and Bruch's membrane, in addition to subretinal and intraretinal vessels. Fluid is always present around the lesion. Alterations, irregularities, and thickening of the ellipsoid zone are always seen. The neuroepithelium is also involved, with the presence of diffuse and cystoid edema. Structural OCT can demonstrate fibrovascular tissue layers under the elevated epithelium.

OCT Angiography Features

Initially located under the pigment epithelium, the new vessels spread out into the outer retinal avascular area, breaking through the pigmented epithelium. The neovascular network is generally extensive and the flow is high. The morphology is varied as the ramifications take on different aspects: new vessels in the shape of a medusa-head, coral, bicycle-wheel, fan, dead tree, tangled network and vascular loop. The overall appearance is clearly different from normal vascularization.

The density of the capillaries may be packed or sparse, the vessels may appear thin and numerous, or, as a result of arterialization and following repeated relapses, they may be thicker, straighter, and rigid, with disappearance of the thinner capillaries.

The loops are mainly present in the periphery of the CNV and they contribute to the formation of new vessels in the shape of a bicycle-wheel, fan or coral. They may be frequent, rare and thin, or dense and fibrillar.

OCT angiography makes it possible to separate the various vascular layers that form the Type 4 new vessels and to specify their characteristics.

1. *Superficial layer or layers:* The Type 2 classical new vessels appear as rounded or fan-shaped, with a feeder vessel that may be highlighted as the point of origin of many thin radial vessels forming loops. Loops are most frequently found in the periphery of the CNV. The assessment of new vessels, a few microns deeper, frequently demonstrates a feeder trunk arising from the choroid.
2. *Deeper layer or layers:* By performing a deeper scan, underneath the pigment epithelium, but above Bruch's membrane, only one or a few Type 1 neovascular membranes are visible. These extend out more widely, and are irregular. They have numerous thicker, and more irregular loops, and are associated with one or more feeder trunks.

A dark halo is consistently seen around these new vessels and is attributed to morphological variations of the choriocapillaris, a screen effect or alteration of the blood flow in the choriocapillaris.

Fluid is always present, resulting in flat detachment of the pigment epithelium and associated with fibrovascular content, detachment of the neuroepithelium and diffuse or cystoid edema. The neovascular complex always includes a feeder trunk or a bundle of feeder vessels (**Figs 7.11 and 7.12**).

NEOVASCULAR MEMBRANES IN MYOPIA

These neovascular membranes develop above the pigmented epithelium. They may penetrate into the external avascular retinal area. These are typically Type 2 classical new vessels and are almost always small in size.

Clinical Features

The neovascular membranes are roundish and gray in appearance, without intraretinal or subretinal pooling of fluid. There are neither any signs of pigment epithelium detachment nor edema. Occasionally there are hemorrhages. If left untreated the new vessels grow slowly and their progression is always slower than progression that occurs with Type 1 or Type 2 new vessels.

Fluorescein Angiography Features

The myopic Type 2 new vessels are smaller than Type 1 new vessels. Hyperfluorescence is initially punctiform and widens with dye leakage. Fluorescein angiography in these cases is affected by dye leakage preventing the observation of the structure of the vascular membrane.

Structural OCT Features

A roundish or spindle-shaped hyper-reflective area can be noticed along the CNV margin. Retina may be thicker and the neuroepithelium is invariably involved. Cystoid or diffuse edema is seldom seen.

OCT Angiography Features

The myopic neovascular membrane has a glomerular or globular aspect, and within the membrane, the capillaries are convoluted and tangled. The membrane forms an irregular globe with apparently sharp boundaries and a pseudo-

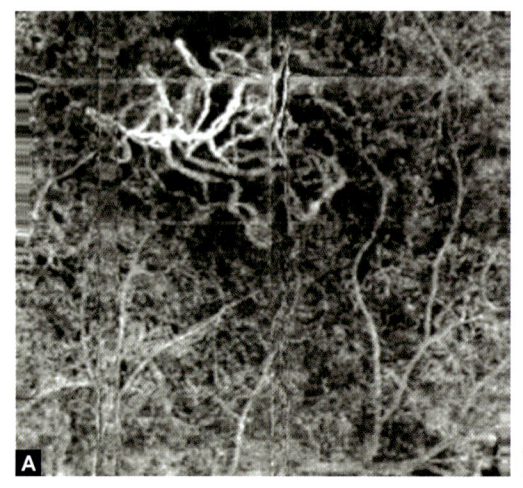

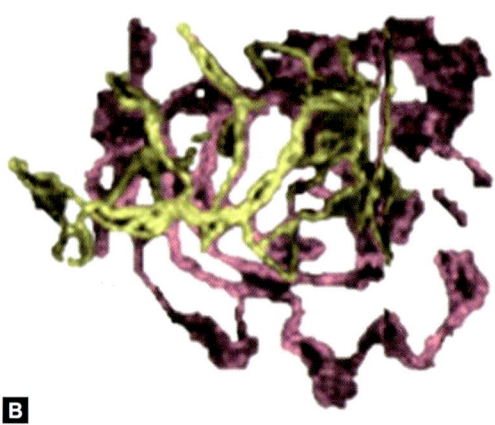

Figures 7.11A and B OCT angiography. Type 4 new vessels: OCT angiography enables identification and description of the separate vascular layers that form the Type 4 new vessels. Type 2 classical new vessels have a rounded, fan-like shape with a feeder vessel from which many thin radial vessels take origin and form loops at the periphery

Type 1, Type 2 and Type 4 (Mixed) Choroidal Neovascularization | 53

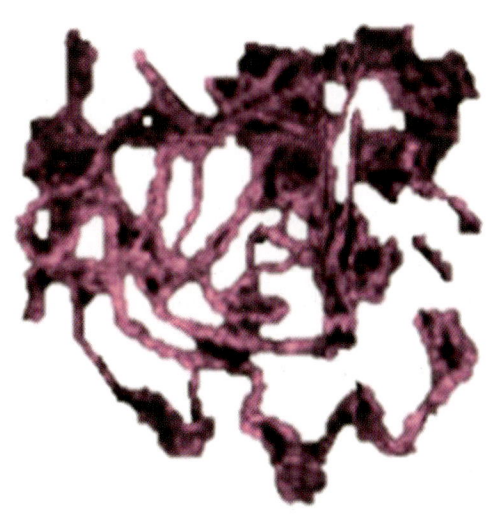

Figure 7.12 OCT angiography. Type 4 new vessels: OCT angiography makes it possible to highlight the various vascular layers. By performing a deeper study, beneath the pigment epithelium but above the Bruch's membrane, a much more extensive Type 1 neovascular membrane can be identified with many thicker and more irregular branches and loops, and one or more feeder trunks. There is always a dark halo around the new vessels attributed to morphological alterations of the choriocapillaris, a screen effect or alterations of the blood flow in the choriocapillaris

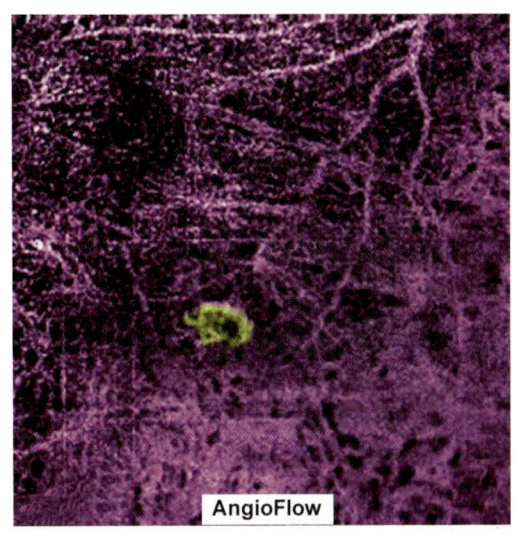

Figure 7.14 OCT angiography. Myopic new vessels: In rarer cases, as seen here, the membrane is large in size and appears to have sharp boundaries. The newly formed capillaries are tangled and convoluted with a dense capillary network

Table 7.8 Morphology of myopic CNV
Generally
• Tuft shaped • Glomerular shaped • Globular
Rarely
• Medusa head • Coral shaped

Abbreviation: CNV, choroidal neovascularization

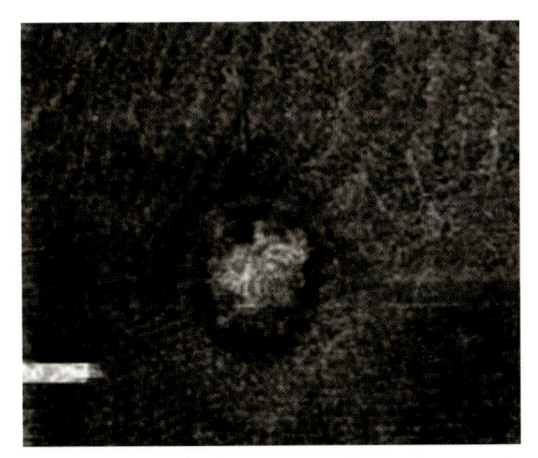

Figure 7.13 OCT angiography. Glomerular myopic new vessels: The myopic neovascular membrane has a glomerular, globular appearance, with convoluted, tangled capillaries within. The membrane forms an irregular globe with apparently sharp boundaries and a pseudoencapsulated appearance

encapsulated appearance. Occasionally, the CNV is tuft shaped **(Table 7.8)**.

More seldom the membrane is large and seems to present sharp boundaries. Rarely the membrane may have a medusa-head or coral-shaped appearance. The newly formed capillaries are tangled and convoluted with a dense capillary network **(Figs 7.13 and 7.14)**.

Fibrotic CNV show rare and thick CNV located inside a fibrous formation **(Figs 7.15 and 7.16)**.

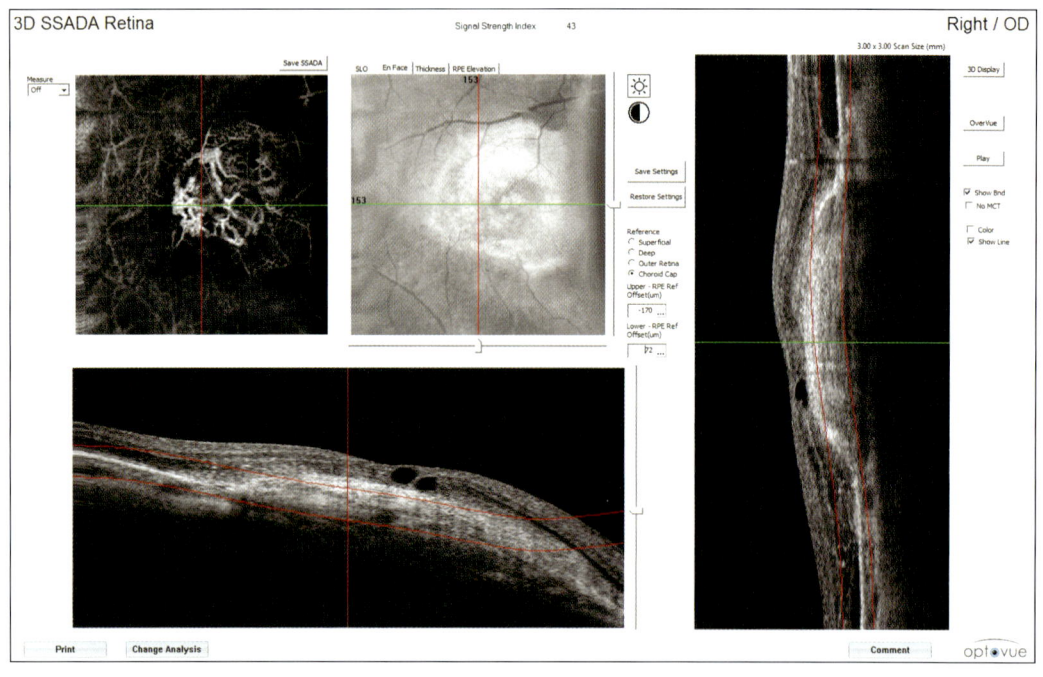

Figure 7.15 Fibrotic membrane with rare thick vessels

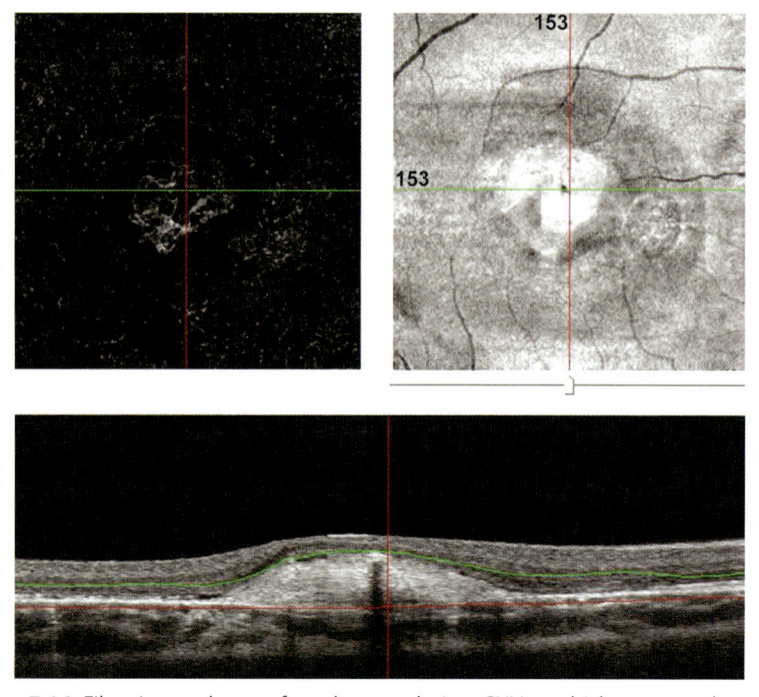

Figure 7.16 Fibrotic membrane after a long evolution, CNV are thick sparse and tangled, located inside a fibrous formation

BIBLIOGRAPHY

1. Kuehlewein L, Dansingani KK, de Carlo TE, et al. Optical coherence tomography angiography of type 3 neovascularization secondary to age-related macular degeneration. Retina. 2015;35(11):2229-35.
2. Kuehlewein L, Sadda SR, Sarraf D. OCT angiography and sequential quantitative analysis of type 2 neovascularization after ranibizumab therapy. Eye (Lond). 2015;29(7):932-5.
3. Lumbroso B, Rispoli M, Savastano MC. Longitudinal optical coherence tomography-angiography study of type 2 naive choroidal neovascularization early response after treatment. Retina. 2015;35(11):2242-51.
4. Mastropasqua R, Di Antonio L, Di Staso S, et al. Optical Coherence Tomography Angiography in Retinal Vascular Diseases and Choroidal Neovascularization. J Ophthalmol. 2015;2015:343515.
5. Spaide RF. Optical Coherence Tomography Angiography Signs of Vascular Abnormalization with Antiangiogenic Therapy for Choroidal Neovascularization. Am J Ophthalmol. 2015; 160(1):6-16.
6. Jia Y, Bailey ST, Wilson DJ, et al. Quantitative optical coherence tomography angiography of choroidal neovascularization in age-related macular degeneration. Ophthalmology. 2014; 121(7):1435-44.

58 | Practical Handbook of OCT Angiography

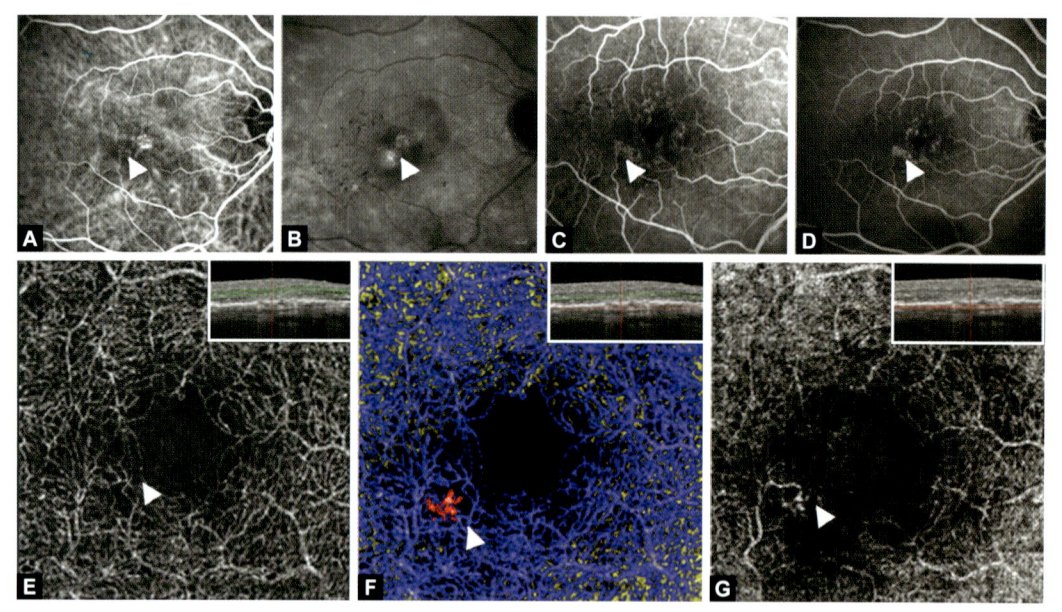

Figures 8.3A to G Multimodal imaging of the RE of an 80-year-old female diagnosed with Type 3 neovascularization treated by 3 intravitreal anti-VEGF injections: (A) Early frame of indocyanine green angiography (ICGA) shows the presence of a hypercyanescent lesion (arrowhead) at the border of the foveal avascular zone (FAZ); (B) Late frames of ICGA show the presence of a typical "hot spot" (arrowhead) in the perifoveal region; (C) Very early frames of fluorescein angiography (FA) show a small hyperfluorescent lesion (arrowhead), corresponding to an intense hyperfluorescence in the late frames of FA (D); (E), (F) and (G) 3 x 3 mm optical coherence tomographic angiography (OCT-A) images with correlating optical coherence tomography (OCT) B-scan; (E) OCT-A, deep capillary plexus segmentation shows a discrete round lesion (arrowhead); (F) Stacked color image of the outer retinal segmentation reveals a high-flow lesion, which seems to extend downwards into the choriocapillaris (G), giving rise to a tuft-shaped lesion in the narrow segmentation corresponding to a 30-microns area around the Bruch's membrane (arrowhead). Note the projection artifact of superficial capillary plexus (blue on the stacked color image) on (F) and (G)

giving rise to a hot spot in indocyanine green angiography (ICGA) late frames **(Figs 8.1 to 8.4)**.[4,8,9]

The advent of OCT angiography (OCT-A) allowed an in-depth analysis of retinal microcirculation, giving interesting insights into this peculiar vascular complex. In OCT-A, type 3 neovascularization is characterized by a retinal-retinal anastomosis that emerges from the deep capillary plexus **(Figs 8.1 to 8.4)**, forming a *tuft-shaped* high-flow network **(Figs 8.2 and 8.3)** in the outer retinal segmentation, and finally abutting in the sub-RPE space. Further, the tuft-shaped lesion corresponds to a *small glomerular-shaped* **(Figs 8.2 to 8.4)** lesion in the choriocapillaris segmentation. However, this glomerular lesion appears to be connected with the choroid through a small caliber vessel only in a minority of cases. Thus, OCT-A confirms the hypothesis that in a majority of cases the early appearance of Type 3 neovascularization is characterized by an intra-retinal vascular complex emanating from the deep capillary plexus. Moreover, the intraretinal proliferation may be associated with evolving sub-RPE neovascular tissue, corresponding to the small glomerular lesion in the choriocapillaris segmentation on OCT-A images.

Based on these features, OCT-A may be considered as a very reliable imaging technique for the detection, diagnosis and monitoring of these small, high flows, peculiar intraretinal lesions. Scanning areas of 2 × 2 or 3 × 3 mm and

Type 3 Neovascularization Features on Optical Coherence Tomography Angiography

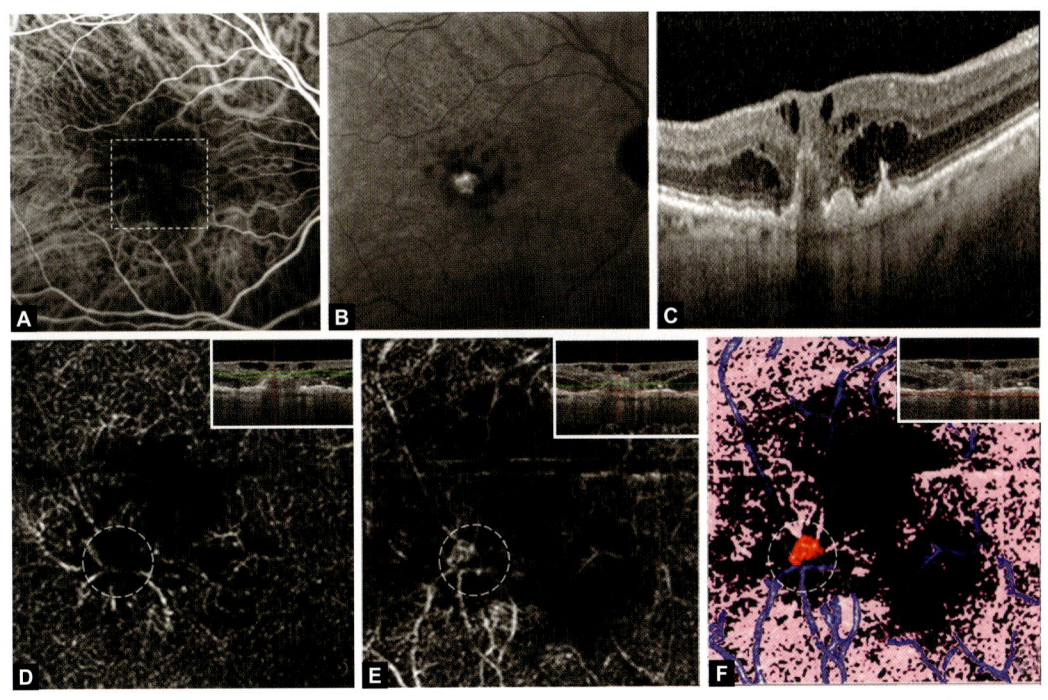

Figures 8.4A to F Multimodal imaging of the LE of a 79-year-old female diagnosed with Type 3 neovascularization, previously treated by 6 intravitreal anti-VEGF injections: (A) Early frame of indocyanine green angiography (ICGA) shows the connection between a third order arteriole and venule at the border of the foveal avascular zone (FAZ); (B) Late frames of ICGA show the presence of a typical "hot spot"; (C) B-scan demonstrates a focal funnel-shaped defect in the RPE accompanied by subretinal and intraretinal fluid; (D), (E) and (F) 2 x 2 mm optical coherence tomographic angiography (OCT-A) images with correlating optical coherence tomography (OCT) B-scan; (E) OCT-A deep capillary plexus segmentation showing two high-flow vessels extending posteriorly, surrounded by black, no-flow, no-signal cystic spaces (dotted circle); (F) The outer retinal segmentation reveals a high flow plexiform lesion (dotted circle), which seems to drag downwards (stacked color image on G), giving further rise to a plexiform lesion (red on the stacked color image) in the narrow segmentation corresponding to a 30-microns area around the Bruch's membrane (dotted circle). Deeper segmentation reveals the presence of a corresponding glomerular lesion

an appropriate segmentation of the deep capillary plexus, outer retinal layers and choriocapillaris provide an interesting insight into the pathophysiology and evolution of these lesions.

REFERENCES

1. Freund KB, Ho IV, Barbazetto IA, et al. Type 3 neovascularization: the expanded spectrum of retinal angiomatous proliferation. Retina. 2008;28:201-11.
2. Gass JD. Stereoscopic Atlas of Macular Diseases, 4th edn. St. Louis, MO. CV Mosby; 1997. pp. 26-30.
3. Gass JD. Biomicroscopic and histopathologic considerations regarding the feasibility of surgical excision of subfoveal neovascular membranes. Am J Ophthalmol. 1994;118:258-98.
4. Querques G, Souied EH, Freund KB. How has high-resolution multimodal imaging refined our understanding of the vasogenic process in type 3 neovascularization? Retina. 2015;35:603-13.

CHOROIDAL NEW VESSEL COMPLICATIONS IN MULTIFOCAL CHOROIDITIS

Multifocal choroiditis (MC) is an inflammatory disease, which leaves numerous small scars on the fundus in its scar phase. On fluorescein angiography, scars of choroiditis are generally hyperfluorescent without late-stage dye diffusion during the sequence. This appearance contrasts with early hyperfluorescence and late-stage leakage seen in visible CNV, which can complicate the inflammatory disease. On indocyanine green angiography, the scars are hypocyanescent and their visualization depends on the size and the state of perfusion of the choriocapillaris. The CNV are often hypercyanescent at the center, and hypofluorescent or of average fluorescence at the peripheral fringe. On OCT angiography, the visible neovascular network is comprised of several large trunks anastomosing by vascular loops within the membrane, as well as at its periphery (**Figs 9.13 and 9.14**).

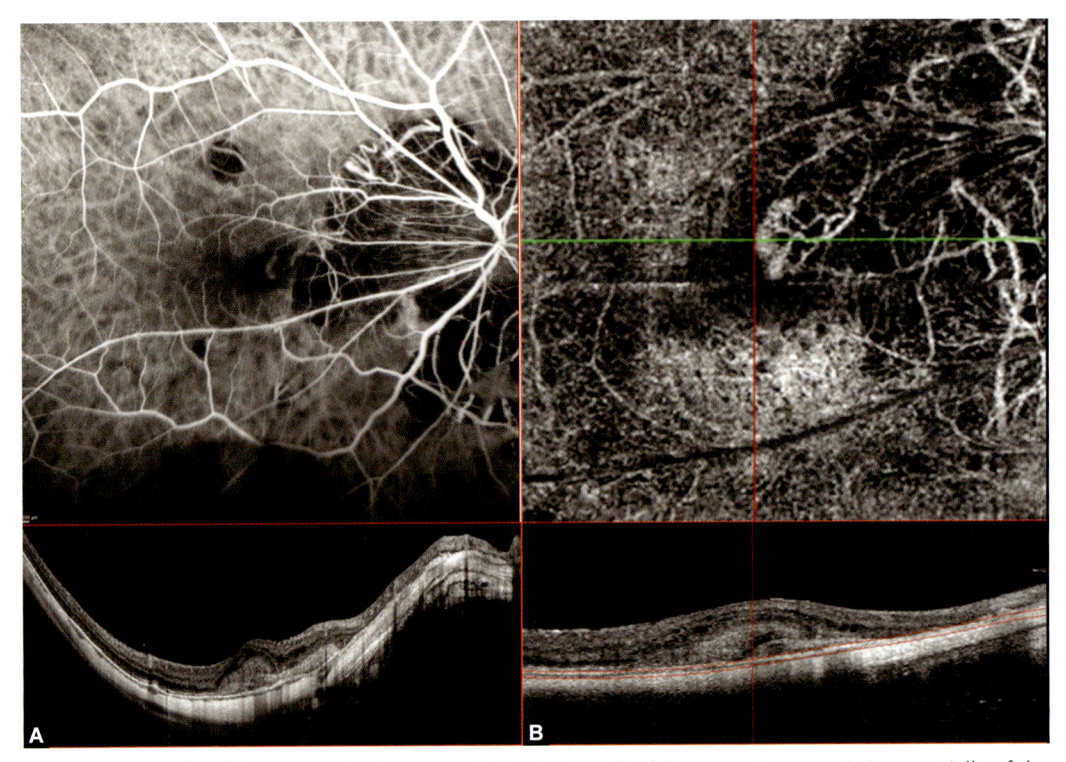

Figures 9.1A and B (A) The choroidal neovascularization (CNV) of degenerative myopia is essentially of the visible type (Type 2). The neovascular network is not clearly visible on fluorescein angiography (FA) owing to the small size of the neovascular membranes. On optical coherence tomography (OCT) B-scan, the subretinal exudation is often scanty and the pre-epithelial CNV are seen as hyper-reflective intraretinal material. Above the retinal pigment epithelium (RPE), it is possible to identify the "hyper-reflective gray" in connection with the exudate and the hyper-reflective subretinal material corresponding to the neovascular membrane; (B) The high sensitivity and specificity of OCT angiography allows very precise visualization of small-sized neovascular membranes. The large neovascular trunks are contrasted against the hypoperfused background. This hypoperfused area associated with visible CNV (hypoperfusion or masking linked to exudation) shows choroidal changes. The peripheral neovascular fringe made up of finer, immature vessels is visible as a slightly blurred decorrelation signal as the CNV-related edema results in optical attenuation of the signal

Choroidal Neovascularization in Diseases other than Age-related Macular Degeneration | **63**

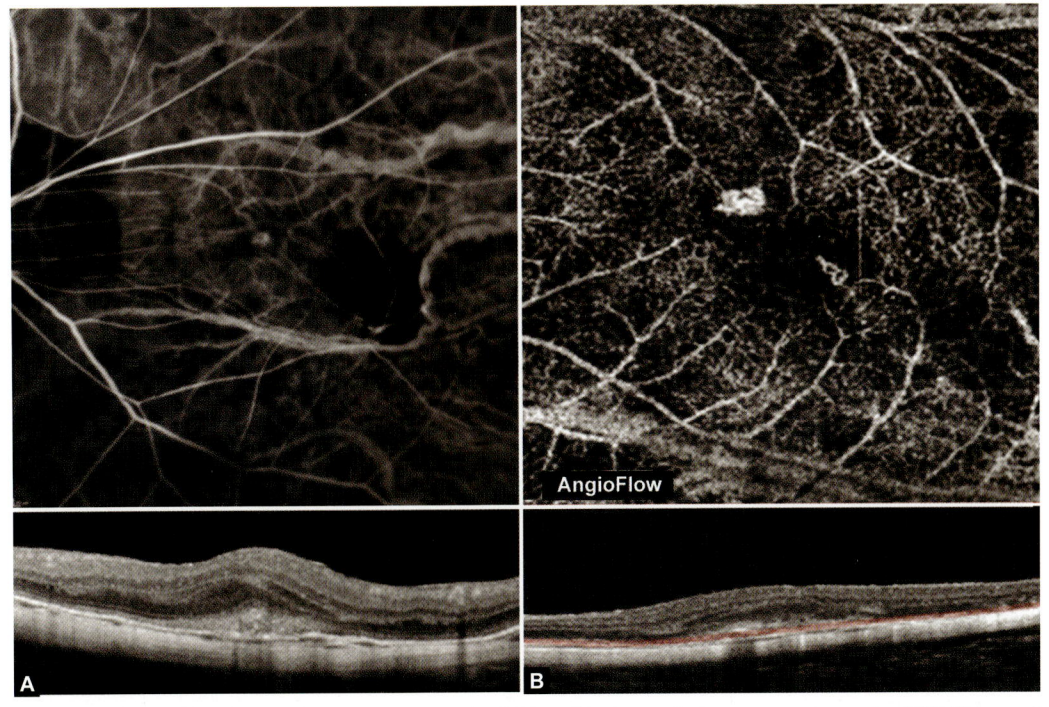

Figures 9.2A and B (A) Fluorescein angiography (FA) and indocyanine green angiography (ICG-A) cannot reliably detect details of vascular architecture in degenerative myopia owing to the small size of the vessels; (B) OCT angiography (3 mm × 3 mm cube) easily detects the flow of CNV, visible clearly as a target-shaped appearance. A decorrelation signal can be seen inferotemporally to the fovea that corresponds to a small zone of atrophy in the bed of a Bruch's membrane rupture, resulting in a "window effect"

64 Practical Handbook of OCT Angiography

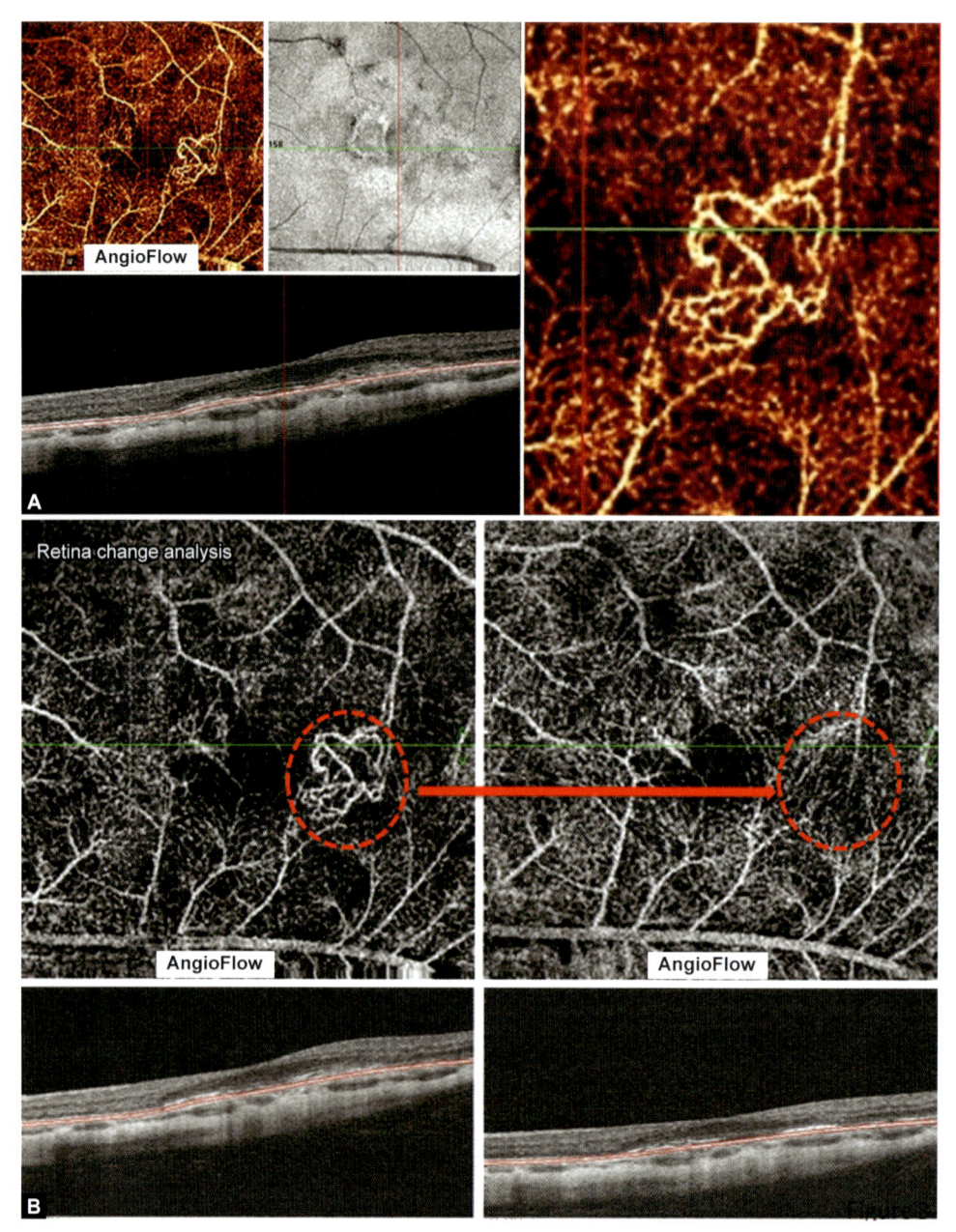

Figures 9.3A and B (A) OCT angiography (3 mm × 3 mm cube). The CNV associated with degenerative myopia is characterized by large anastomosing trunks, linked by loops at the periphery of the membrane. The structure of this CNV is suggestive of recent neovascularization as its vascular density is low. OCT B-scan confirms the presence of active neovascularization characterized by hyper-reflective subretinal material and the associated diffuse edema; (B) Follow-up images of CNV described in (A), before and after anti-VEGF therapy. A single intravitreal injection of anti-VEGF completely eradicated the decorrelation signal at the level of the neovascular membrane. The enhanced response of CNV in myopic individuals to anti-VEGF, with better functional outcomes and longer lasting results compared to age-related macular degeneration (AMD), emphasizes the differences between CNV of high myopia, and of AMD

Choroidal Neovascularization in Diseases other than Age-related Macular Degeneration | **65**

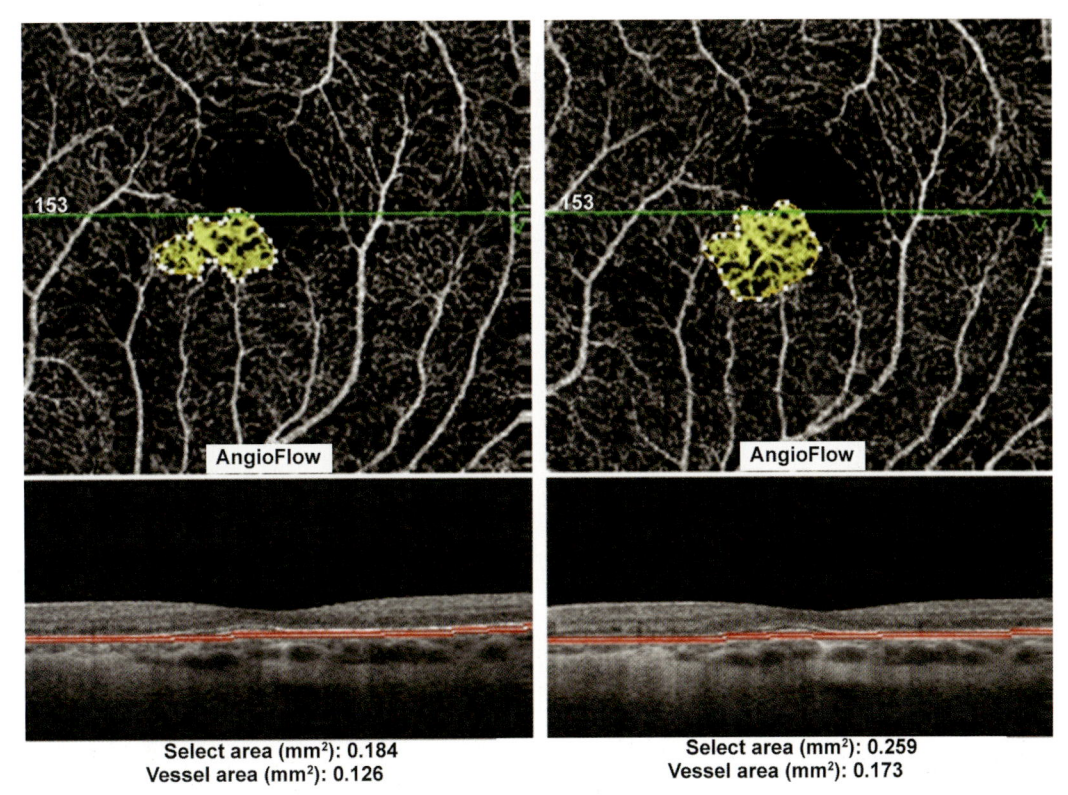

Figure 9.4 Optical coherence tomography (OCT) angiography (3 mm × 3 mm cube). Spontaneous evolution of a neovascular lesion in a young patient with degenerative myopia who refused anti-VEGF treatment. Flow surface measurement software (that enables quantification of involved surface) demonstrates increase in surface of CNV from 0.126 mm² to 0.173 mm² within one month

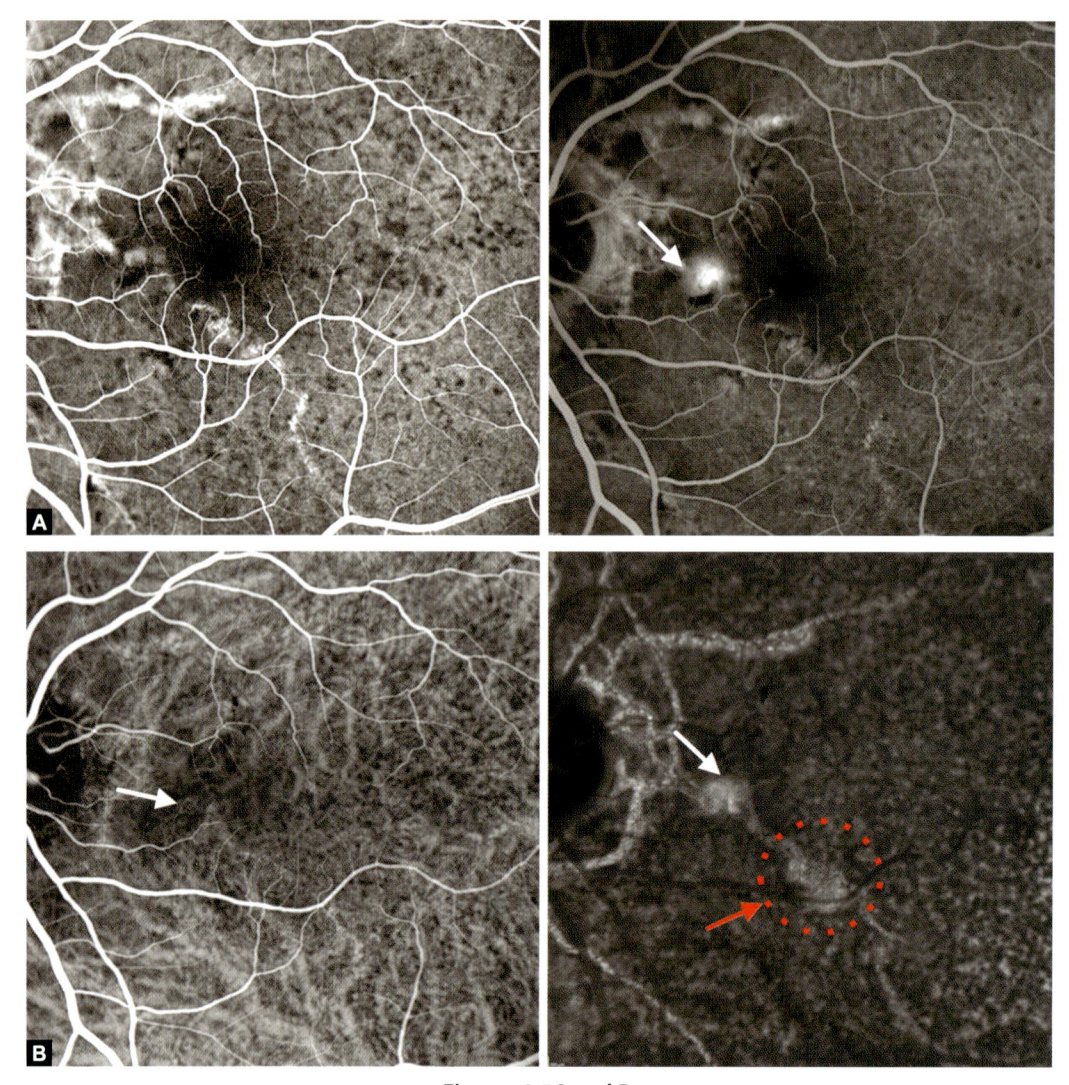

Figures 9.5A and B

Choroidal Neovascularization in Diseases other than Age-related Macular Degeneration | **67**

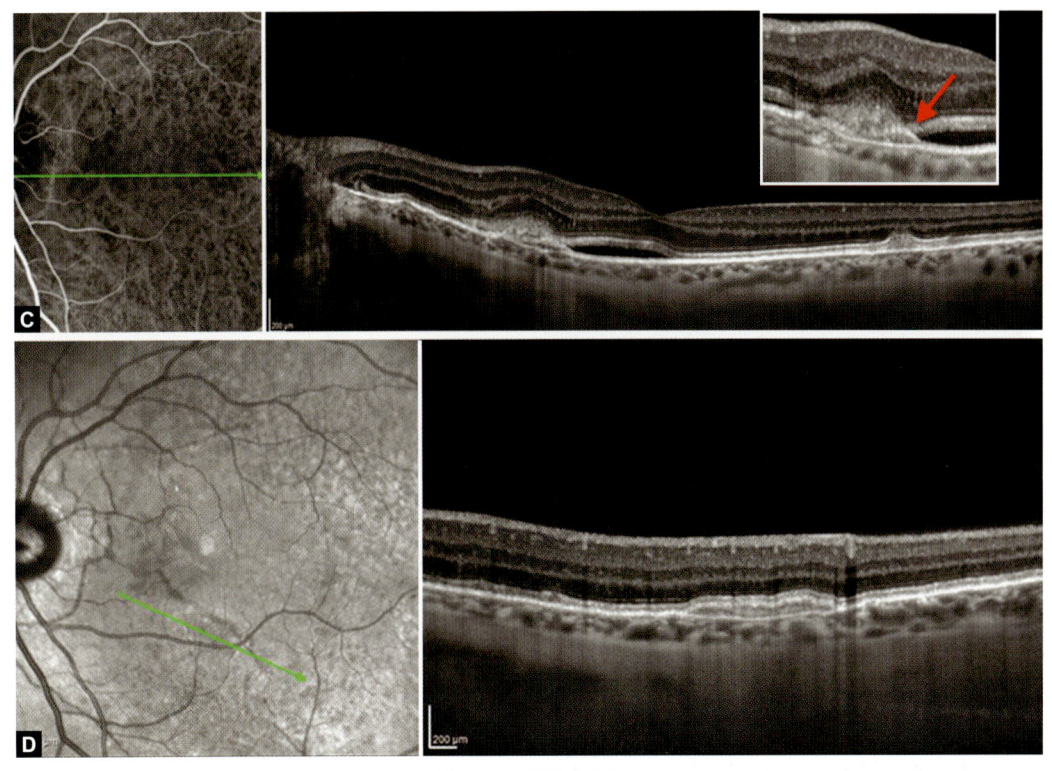

Figures 9.5C and D

Figures 9.5A to D (A) Type 2 CNV are the principal complications in patients with AS. The diagnosis of this complication relies on fluorescein angiography (FA) (white arrow). Early-stage fluorescence of AS are variable and depend on the quality of the RPE; (B) Indocyanine green angiography (ICG-A) can provide complementary information concerning the presence of Type 1 CNV. AS are always hypercyanescent and sprinkled with tiny "pinpoints". With this imaging, hypercyanescent zones are frequently visible next to CNV (white arrow), and along the bed of an AS (red arrow); (C) CNV of AS in OCT B-scan. Cross-sectional images show the presence of subretinal hyper-reflective material corresponding to visible CNV (A), in addition to epithelial elevations with moderate hyper-reflectivity located beneath the RPE (Type 1 CNV); (D) A slight detachment of the pigment epithelium with average, organized subepithelial reflectivity, and no sign of intraretinal exudation, found along the AS at the point where ICG-A delineates a late hypercyanescent plaque, suggesting the possibility of occult CNV

68 | Practical Handbook of OCT Angiography

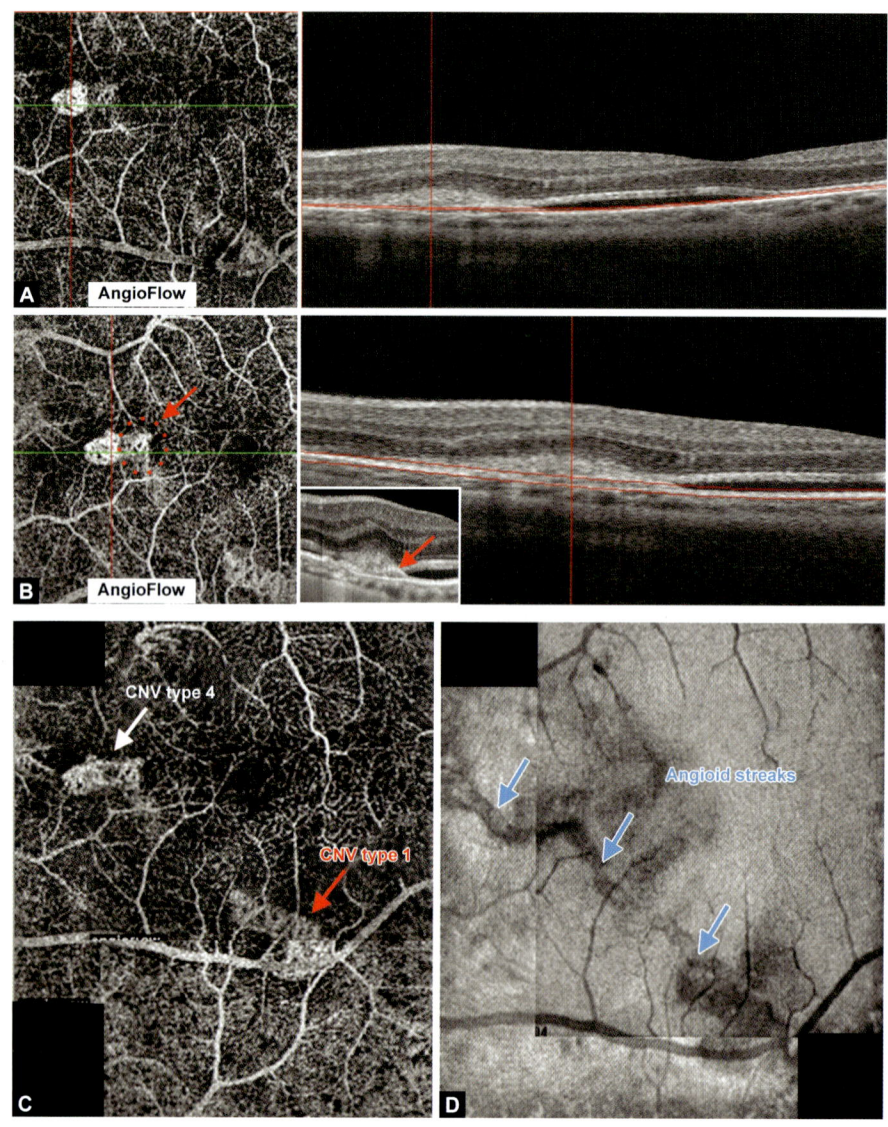

Figures 9.6A to D CNV of AS in OCT angiography (3 mm × 3 mm cube). (A) Type 2 CNV in a "bunched" appearance on cross-section, passing slightly in front of the RPE; (B) Positioning the segmentation lines deep to the RPE allows the occult component of the CNV to be visible. The occult CNV are located near the visible CNV and present a more diffuse and granular decorrelation signal; (C) Composite image of three, 3 mm × 3 mm, cubes with OCT angiography reconstruction of a part of the posterior pole. Note the presence of a decorrelation signal along a streak away from the CNV. This is at the likely location of Type 1 CNV as identified on OCT B-scan, confirmed here by OCT angiography. OCT angiography has made it possible, for the first time, to diagnose mixed CNV within AS and provide a description of the neovascular nature of the hyperfluorescence and hypercyanescence zones; (D) Composite image of three, 3 mm × 3 mm, cubes in *en face* (structural) OCT. The *en face structural* OCT allows visualization of the course of the angioid streaks (darker aspect). It also facilitates the study of the relationship between the streaks and the CNV visualized on OCT angiography. The correlation between structural (*en face OCT*) and functional OCT (OCT angiography) is necessary for an adequate analysis of the information provided by this technique

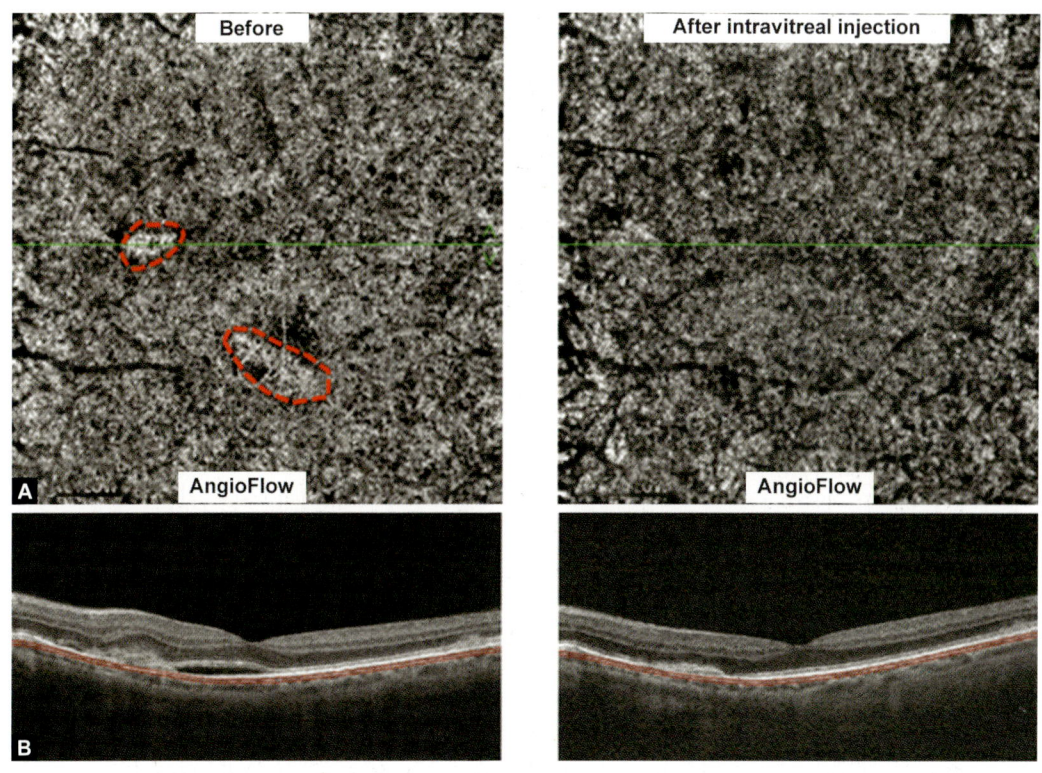

Figures 9.7A and B Follow-up OCT angiography (6 mm × 6 mm cube). CNV of angioid streaks (AS) before and after treatment with anti-VEGF. The decorrelation signals visualized before treatment completely disappear after an intravitreal injection of anti-VEGF, both, in the area corresponding to the visible CNV, as well as in the area of occult CNV

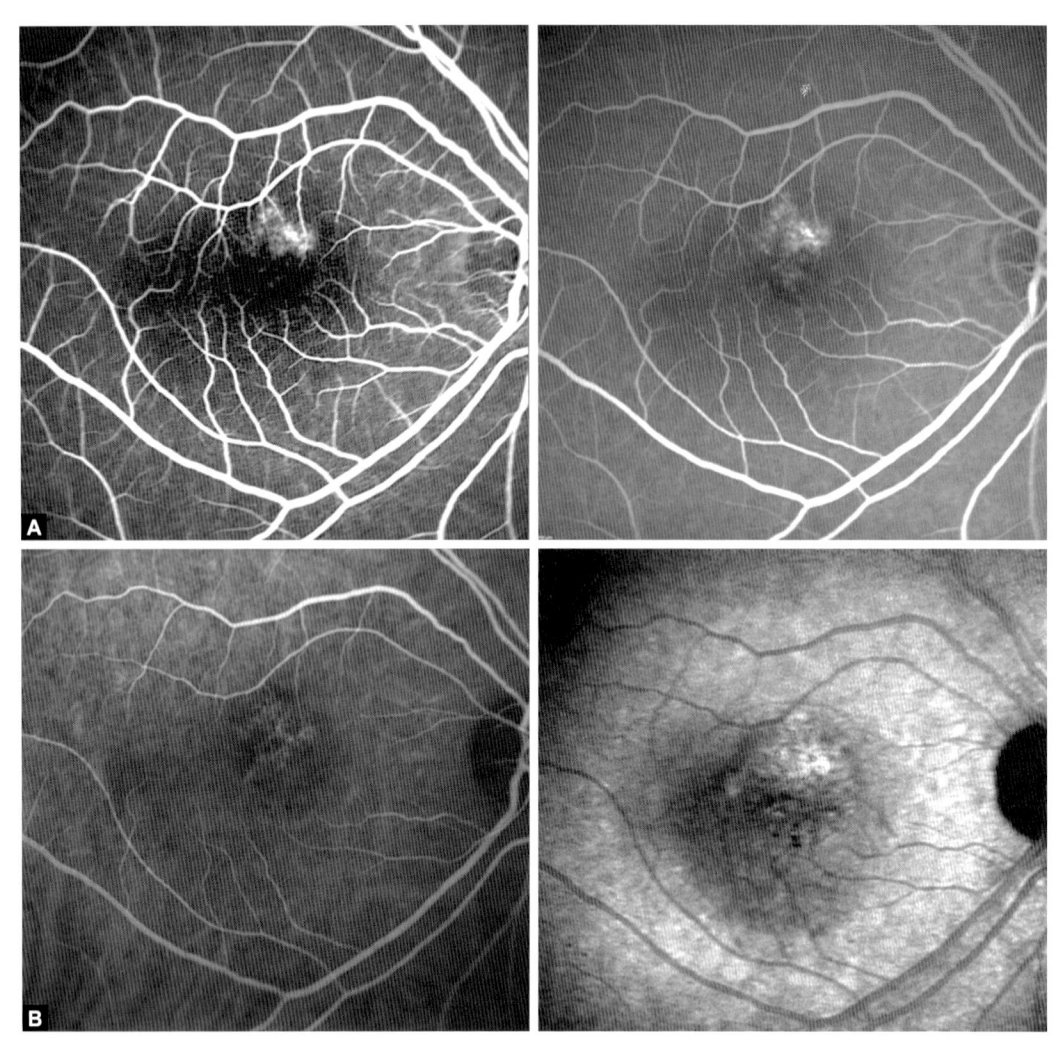

Figures 9.8A and B In cases of chronic central serous chorioretinopathy (CSCR), leakage zones are frequently visible on fluorescein angiography (FA). (A) On indocyanine green angiography (ICG-A); (B) Complications in chronic CSCR, especially when associated with pachychoroid disease, are indicated by the presence of Type 1 choroidal new vessels or by polypoidal choroidal vasculopathy (PCV). Multimodal analysis may fail to give a precise diagnosis or differentiate between these different complications, thus adversely affecting therapy

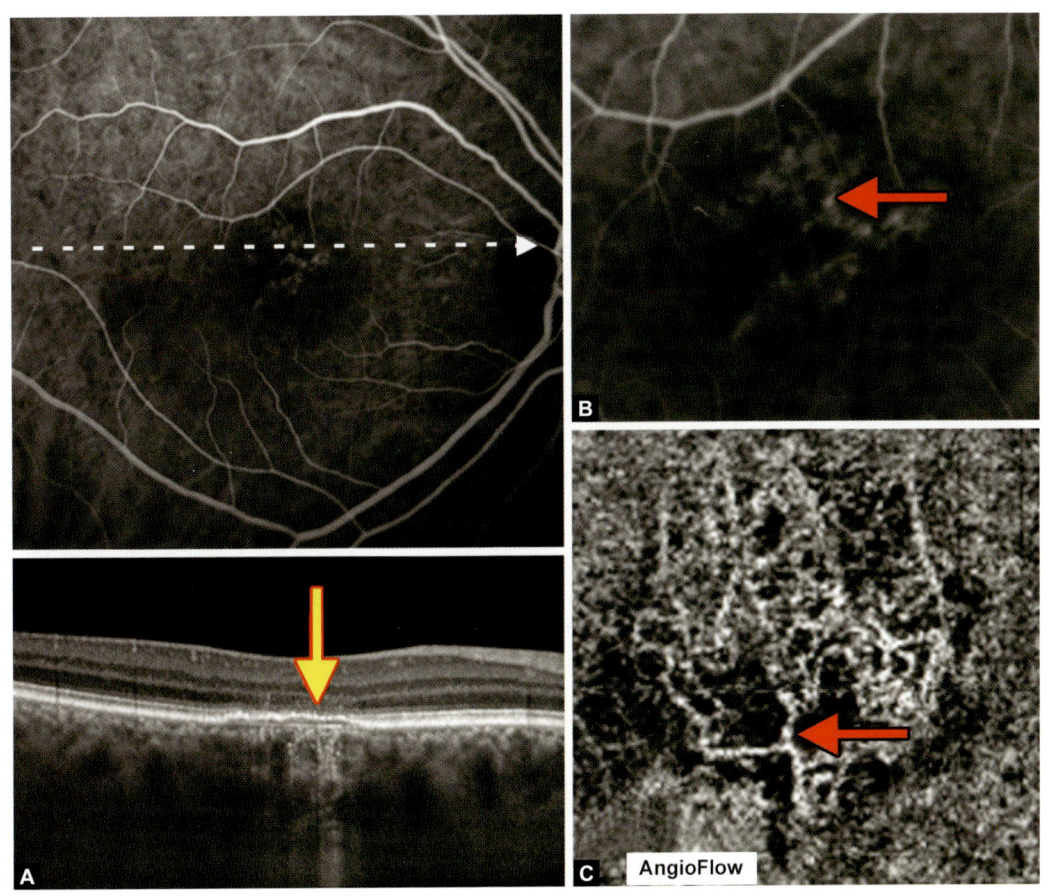

Choroidal Neovascularization in Diseases other than Age-related Macular Degeneration | **71**

Figures 9.9A to C (A) OCT B-scan demonstrates two morphological aspects of the RPE-Bruch's membrane complex. Patients may present with a complex profile that is flat, or lightly detached and undulated with a slight subepithelial reflectivity (yellow arrow); (B) In some cases of chronic CSCR, indocyanine green angiography (ICG-A) aids in the confirmation of suspected CNV. However, the superimposition of several vascular planes makes it difficult to differentiate between CNV and normal choroidal vessels; (C) In OCT angiography, the surface lines with a rather fine slab positioned on the undulated RPE detachment show a Type 1 CNV with fine vascular network and granular decorrelation. The CNV of chronic central serous chorioretinopathy (CSCR) have a structure similar to occult CNV of AMD. The course of some vessels is punctuated by small dilatations, which may be correlated on ICG-A (red arrow)

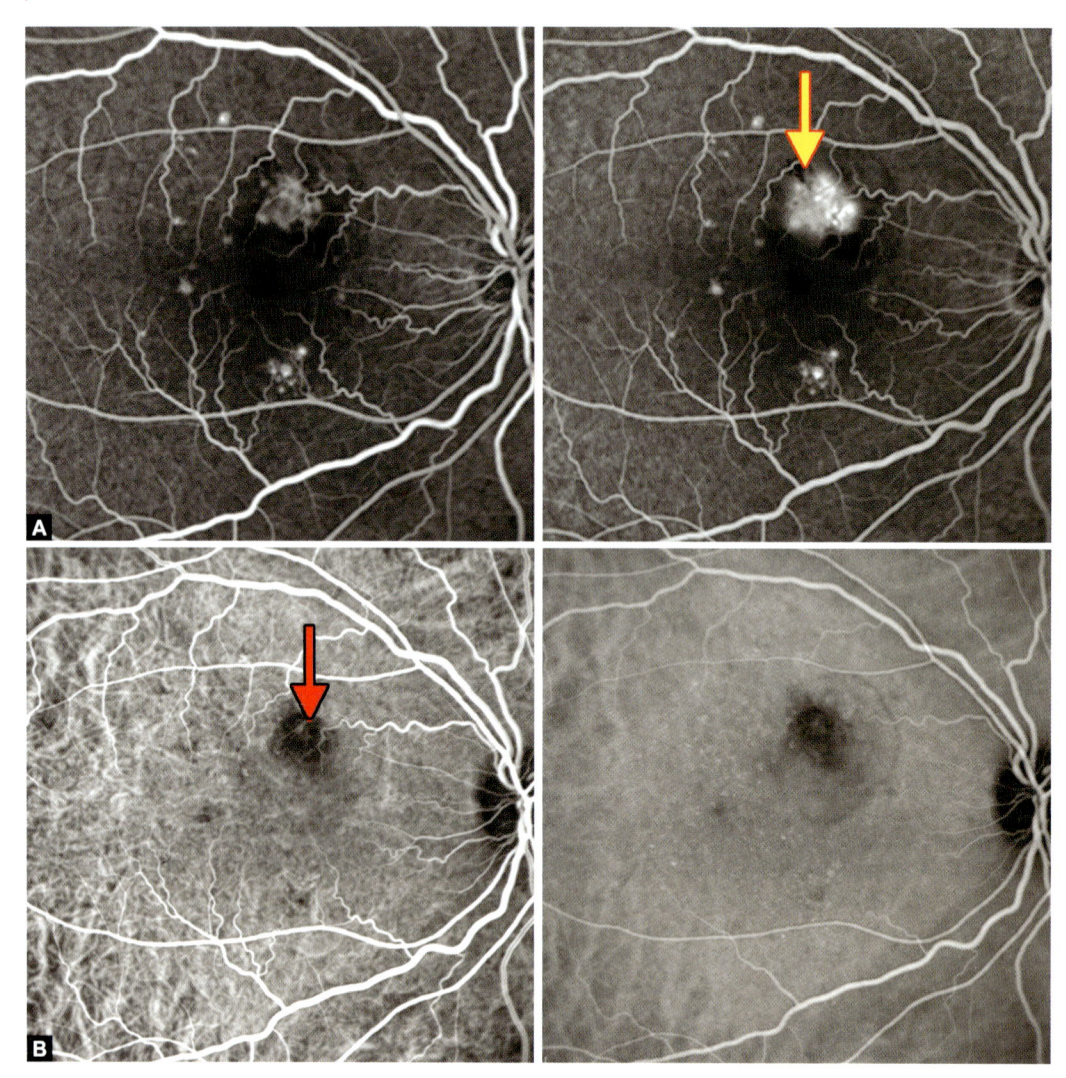

Figures 9.12A and B Multifocal choroiditis (MC) is an inflammatory disease, which leaves numerous small scars on the fundus in its cicatricial phase. (A) On fluorescein angiography (FA), scars of choroiditis are generally hyperfluorescent without late-stage dye diffusion during the sequence. This appearance contrasts with early hyperfluorescence and late-stage leakage seen in visible CNV, which can complicate the inflammatory disease as seen in this case (yellow arrow); (B) On indocyanine green angiography (ICG-A), the scars are hypocyanescent and their visualization depends on the size and the state of perfusion of the choriocapillaris. The CNV are often hypercyanescent at the center, and hypofluorescent or of average fluorescence at the peripheral fringe. "Heart of the membrane" hypercyanescence is associated with the longitudinal visualization of the feeder pedicle (red arrow)

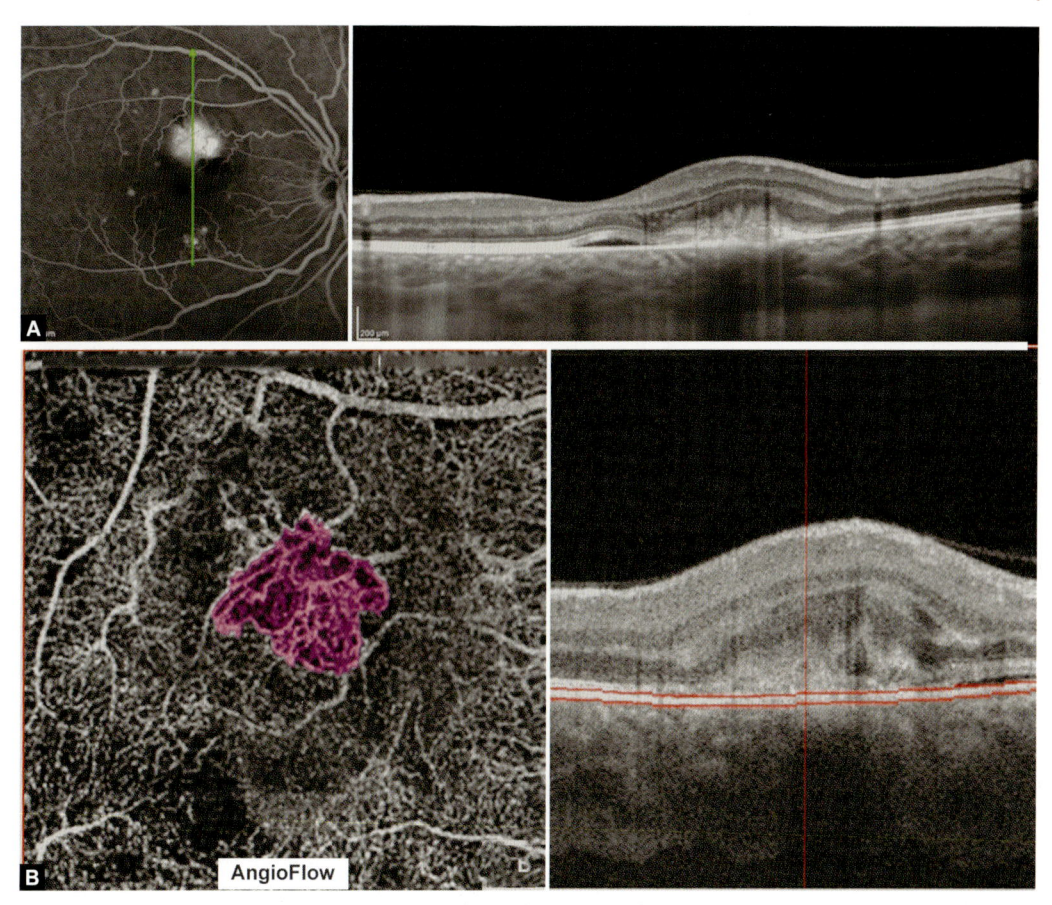

Choroidal Neovascularization in Diseases other than Age-related Macular Degeneration | **75**

Figures 9.13A and B (A) OCT B-scan in CNV of multifocal choroiditis (MC). The CNV appears as a subretinal hyper-reflective zone associated with serous retinal detachment. The continuity of RPE seems altered at the point where the CNV traverse the RPE and pass into the subretinal space; (B) OCT angiography (3 mm × 3 mm cube). The visible neovascular network is comprised of several large trunks anastomosing by vascular loops within the membrane, as well as at its periphery

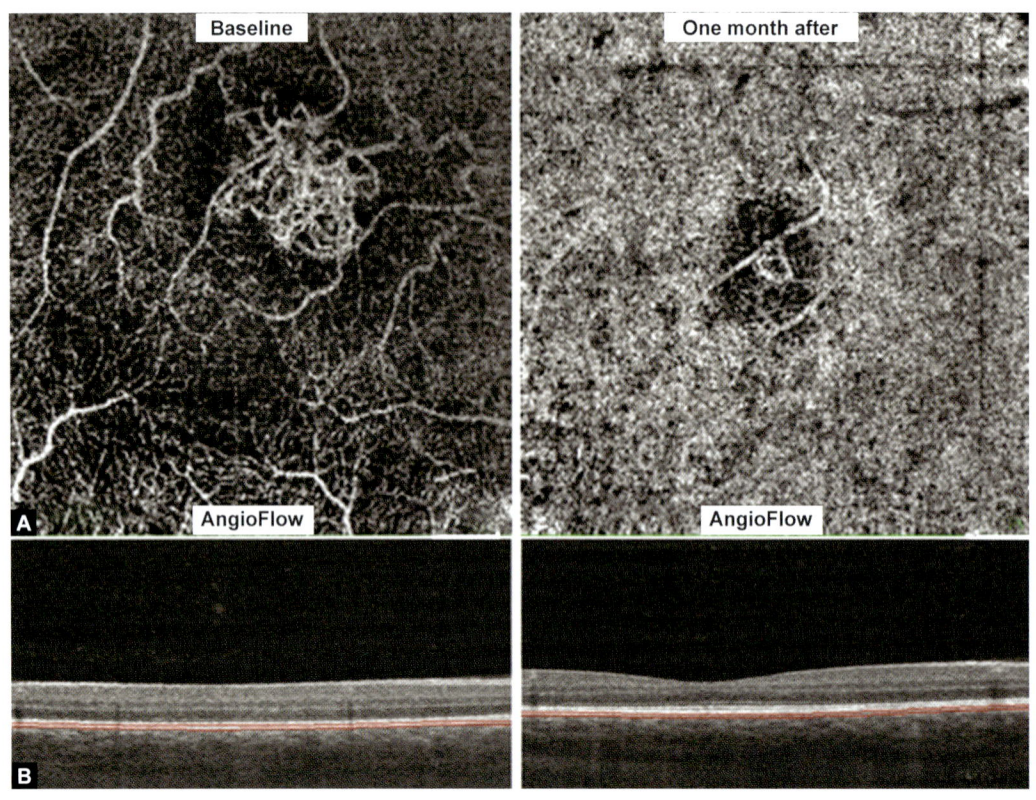

Figures 9.14A and B Follow-up OCT angiography (3 mm × 3 mm cube). The CNV of multifocal choroiditis (MC) on OCT angiography before. (A) After anti-VEGF treatment; (B) The decorrelation signal of the entire peripheral fringe of the CNV disappears after treatment. The only flow that remains is in the feeder pedicle located in the zone where the CNV penetrates the postinflammatory rupture of the RPE. This persistent CNV pedicle may mark the site of possible neovascular recurrences

Choroidal Neovascularization in Diseases other than Age-related Macular Degeneration | 77

POLYPOIDAL CHOROIDAL VASCULOPATHY

Maddalena Quaranta-El Maftouhi, Adil El Maftouhi

Polypoidal choroidal vasculopathy (PCV) is a pathology that includes different entities: idiopathic PCV, PCV secondary to pachychoroid diseases, central serous chorioretinopathy or diffuse retinal epitheliopathy (CSC/DRE), age-related macular degeneration (AMD), and rarer diseases such as tilted disk syndrome, angioid streaks and diseases linked to the presence of a nevus.

Indocyanine green angiography (ICG-A) is the gold standard imaging modality for the diagnosis of PCV. Scanning laser ophthalmoscopy (SLO) angiography is another investigation that enables visualization of the entire lesion. Diseases with PCV have a typical appearance characterized by a branching neovascular network opening out either at the periphery, or within the polypoidal dilations. ICG-A visualization of polypoidal lesions relies on a composite image of fluorescence in different planes and does not depend on their location with respect to the retinal pigment epithelium (RPE).

On the contrary, OCT angiography facilitates segmented analysis of a predefined thickness of tissue at a selected depth. As the entire polypoidal lesion is not located in the same plane, a stratified analysis must be done in order to visualize,

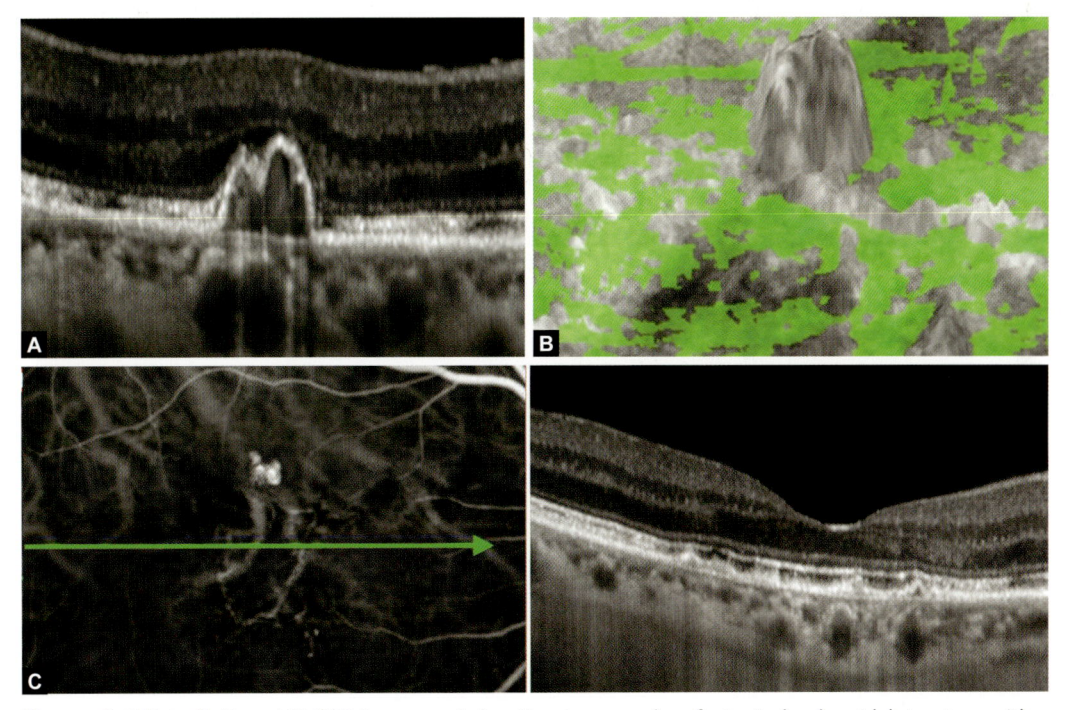

Figures 9.15A to C (A and B) OCT B-scan and elevation topography of a typical polypoidal structure with a pigment epithelial detachment (PED) in the form of a dome with clean, abrupt borders and an olive-shaped subepithelial structure corresponding to polypoidal dilation; (C) The branching network has the appearance of a barely protruding elevation of the epithelium with a slightly wavy profile (double-line sign)

78 | Practical Handbook of OCT Angiography

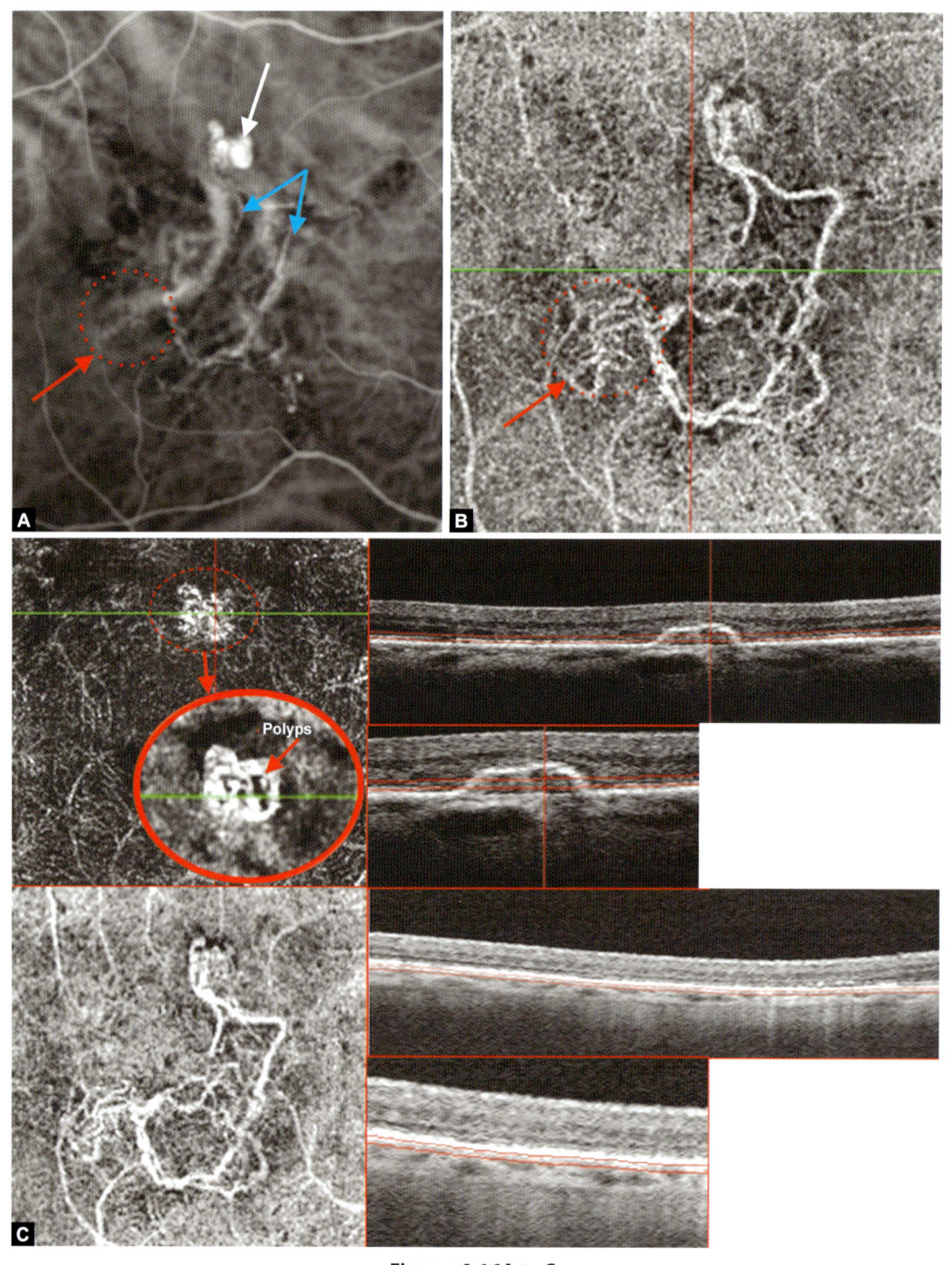

Figures 9.16A to C

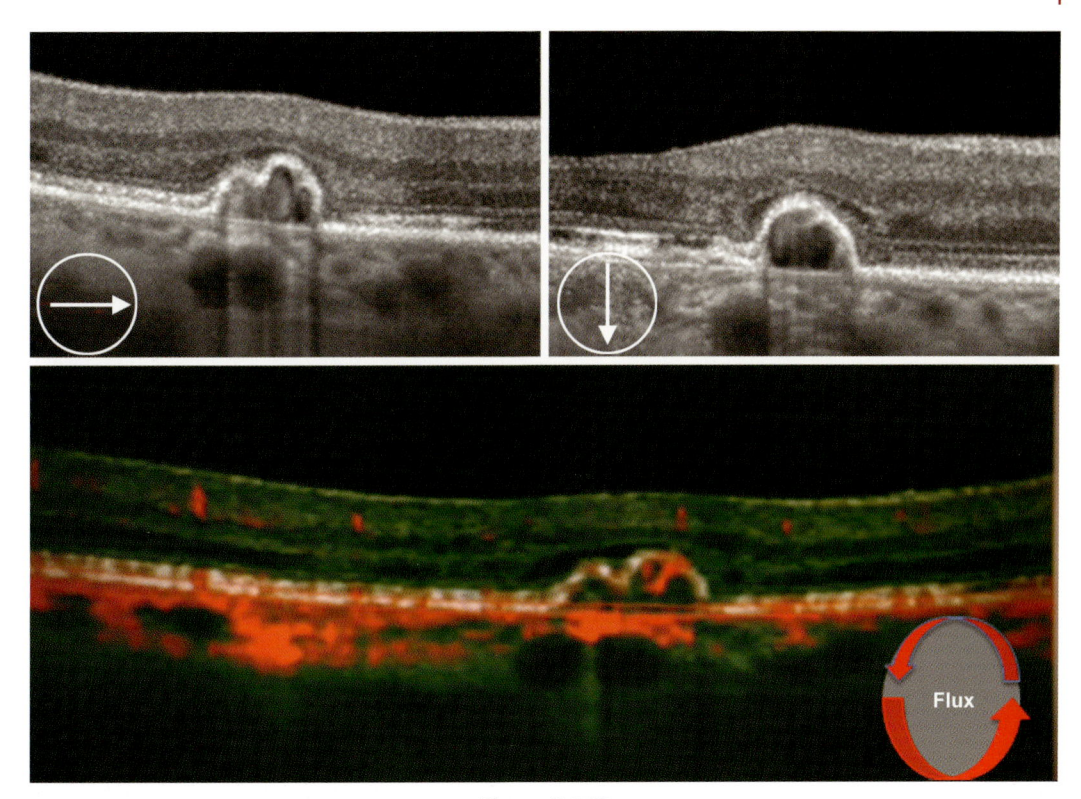

Choroidal Neovascularization in Diseases other than Age-related Macular Degeneration

Figure 9.16D

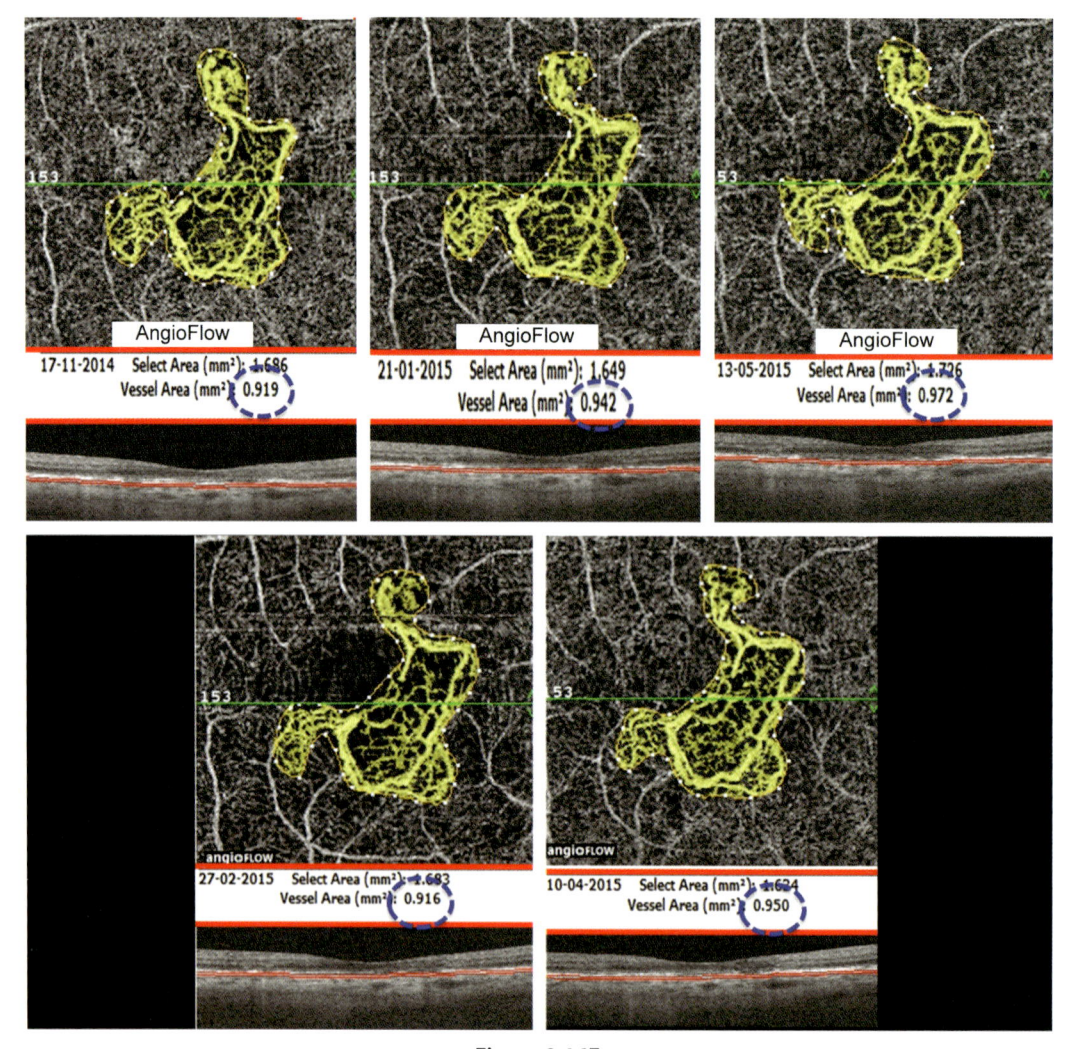

Figure 9.16E

Figures 9.16A to E (A) On ICG angiography, the polyps are visible as early-stage hypercyanescent sacculi (white arrow). Only the main vessels of the interconnecting network are visible (blue arrows) in the early phases of the imaging sequence; (B) On OCT angiography, the branching network is entirely visible in a slab passing underneath the RPE at the level of Bruch's membrane; (C) Visualization of the polyp, which is located in another cross-section, requires positioning the slab in the pigment epithelial detachment (PED); (D) The thickness of the slab must be adapted and maintained proportional to the size of the PED to allow detection of the decorrelation signal corresponding to the polypoidal dilations; (E) Follow-up of the polypoidal lesion during combined treatment with PDT and anti-VEGF. The software program for surface flow provides data for limited modifications of diameter and lesion perfusion despite the disappearance of signs of exudation

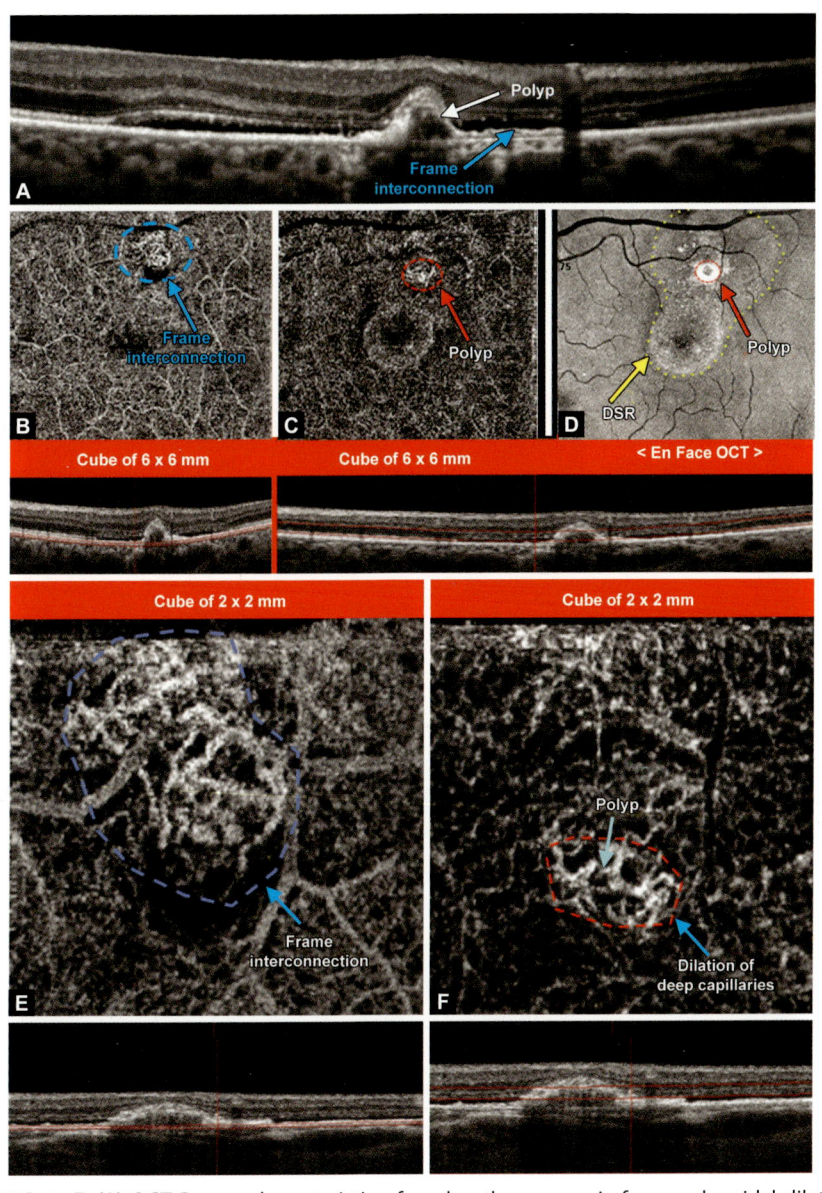

Choroidal Neovascularization in Diseases other than Age-related Macular Degeneration | 81

Figures 9.17A to F (A) OCT B-scan characteristic of, and pathognomonic for, a polypoidal dilation with a serous detachment lamina; (B) OCT angiography (6 mm × 6 mm cube) with a slab positioned at the level of choriocapillaris demonstrating the connective framework of an extrafoveal PCV; (C) OCT angiography (6 mm × 6 mm cube) with a slab positioned at the PED with adapted thickness. The polyps are shown as a decorrelation signal localized along with a part of the interconnecting network; (D) *En face* OCT (structural OCT) combined with OCT angiography provide images of the surface of the retinal serous detachment and polypoidal dilations, which are seen as increased reflectivity around the lesion; (E) OCT angiography (2 mm × 2 mm cube) with a slab positioned at the choriocapillaris level accentuates visualization of the vascular architecture of the interconnecting network; (F) OCT angiography (2 mm × 2 mm cube) with a slab positioned at the PED improves vascular projection and demonstrates the polyp associated with deep capillary dilations by the "magnifying glass" effect

82 Practical Handbook of OCT Angiography

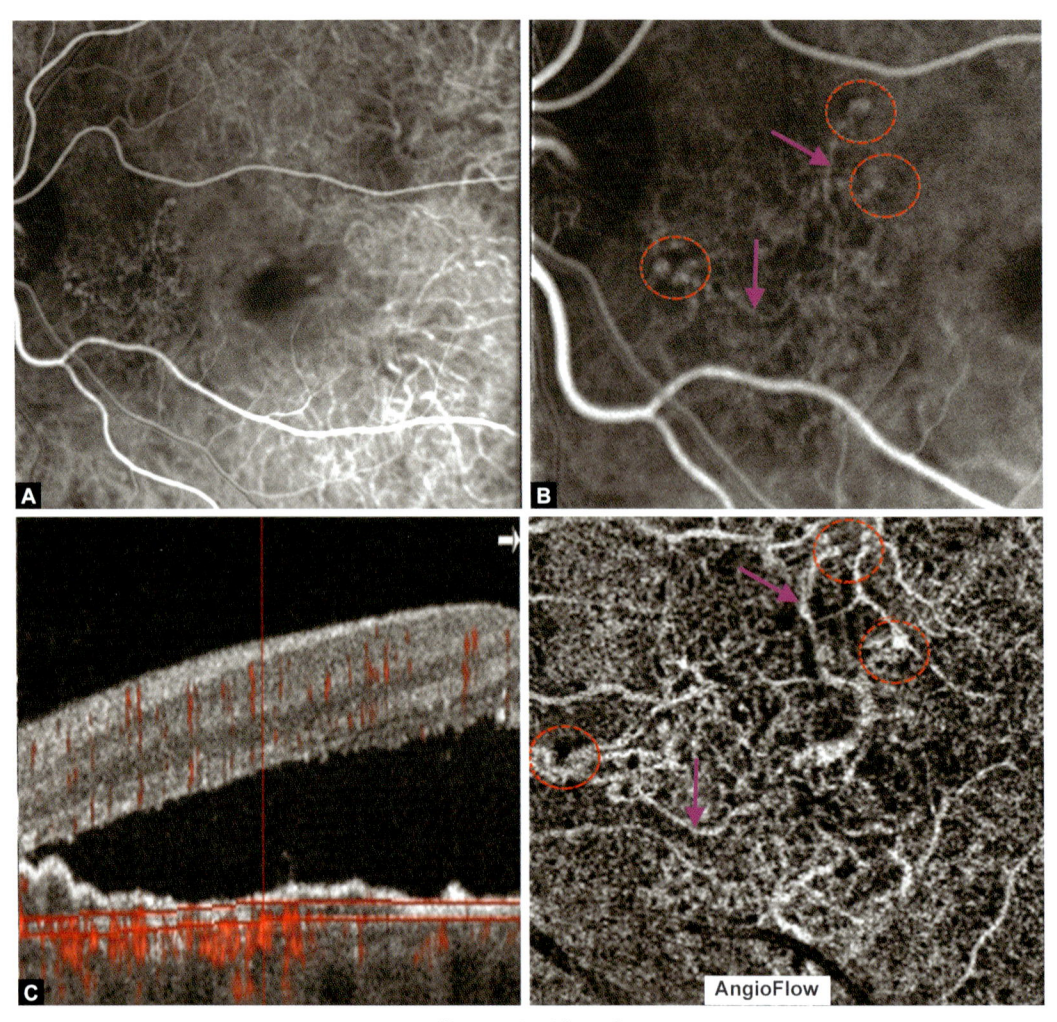

Figures 9.18A to C

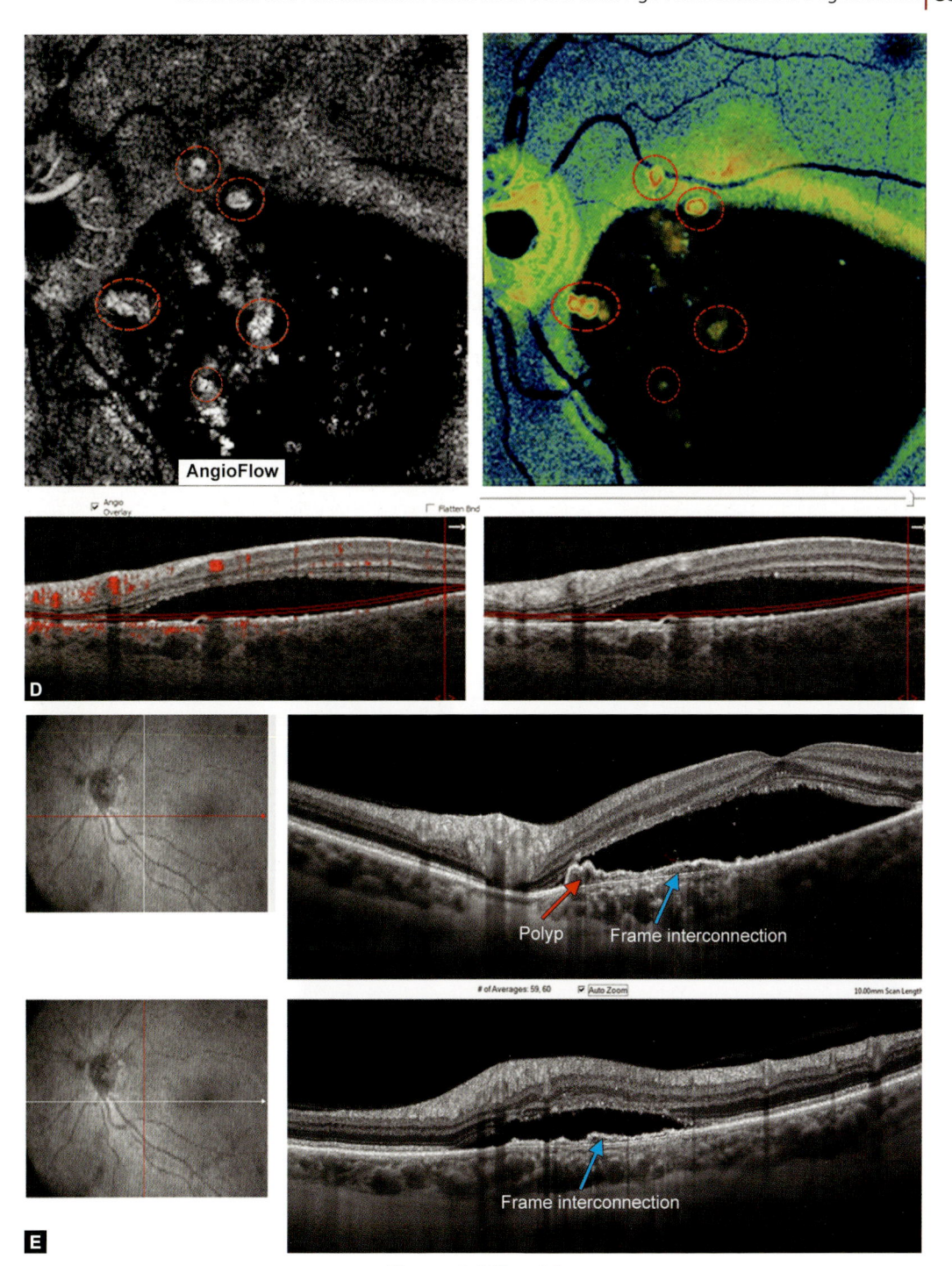

Choroidal Neovascularization in Diseases other than Age-related Macular Degeneration | 83

Figures 9.18D and E

84 | Practical Handbook of OCT Angiography

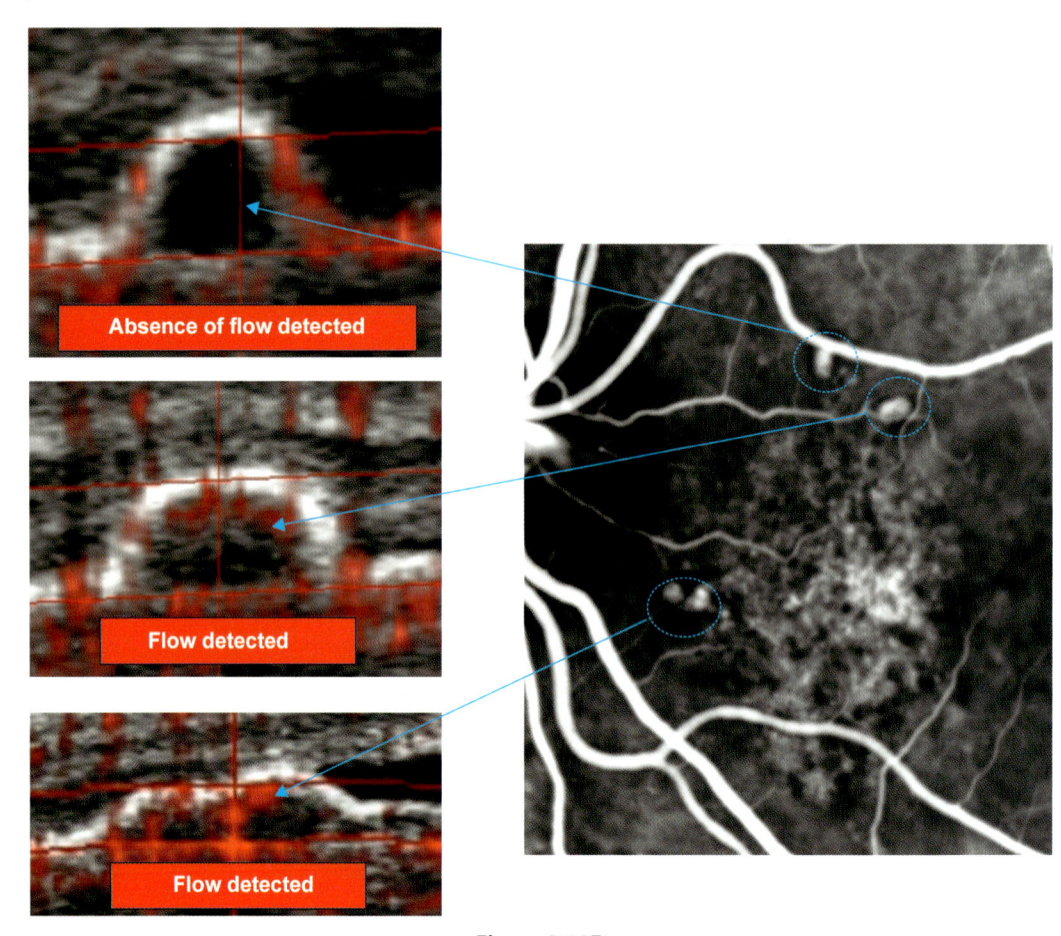

Figure 9.18F

Figures 9.18A to F (A) Early stage of an indocyanine green angiography (ICG-A), which indicates the presence of a very fine connective framework in the interpapillomacular area with polypoidal saccular dilatations; (B) Enlarged view of the interpapillomacular area on ICG-A demonstrating the fine vascular network. The branching network (purple arrows), as well as the polypoidal dilations (red circles) are demonstrated; (C) OCT angiography (3 mm × 3 mm cube). The branching network (purple arrows) is indicated by a segmentation positioned over Bruch's membrane. In contrast, polypoidal dilations (red circles) are barely visible on this slab; (D) OCT angiography (3 mm × 3 mm cube) combined with *en face* OCT with image display in false colors. The thickness and location of the segmentation are modified (in front of Bruch's membrane) in order to better adapt to the PED containing the polyps. The polypoidal dilations on *en face* OCT correspond to the decorrelation signals on OCT angiography. In the second part of the OCT angiography analysis, the polypoidal dilations are more numerous than those seen on ICG-A (red circles); (E) OCT B-scan of the polypoidal lesion demonstrating a relatively flat RPE detachment (neovascular branching network) along with small detachments with abrupt borders (the polyps); (F) Cross section scans showing flow inside the polyps

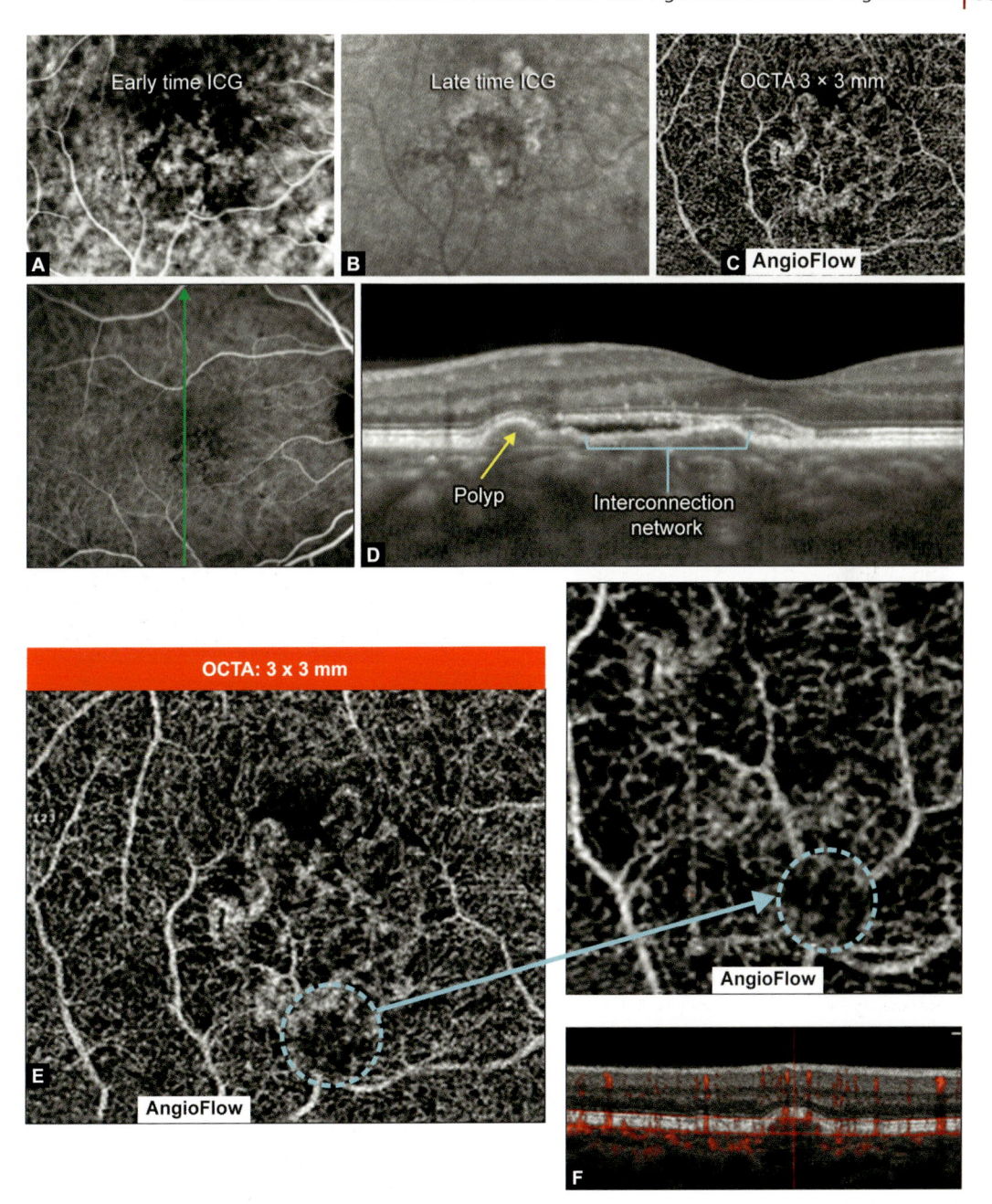

Choroidal Neovascularization in Diseases other than Age-related Macular Degeneration | 85

Figures 9.19A to F

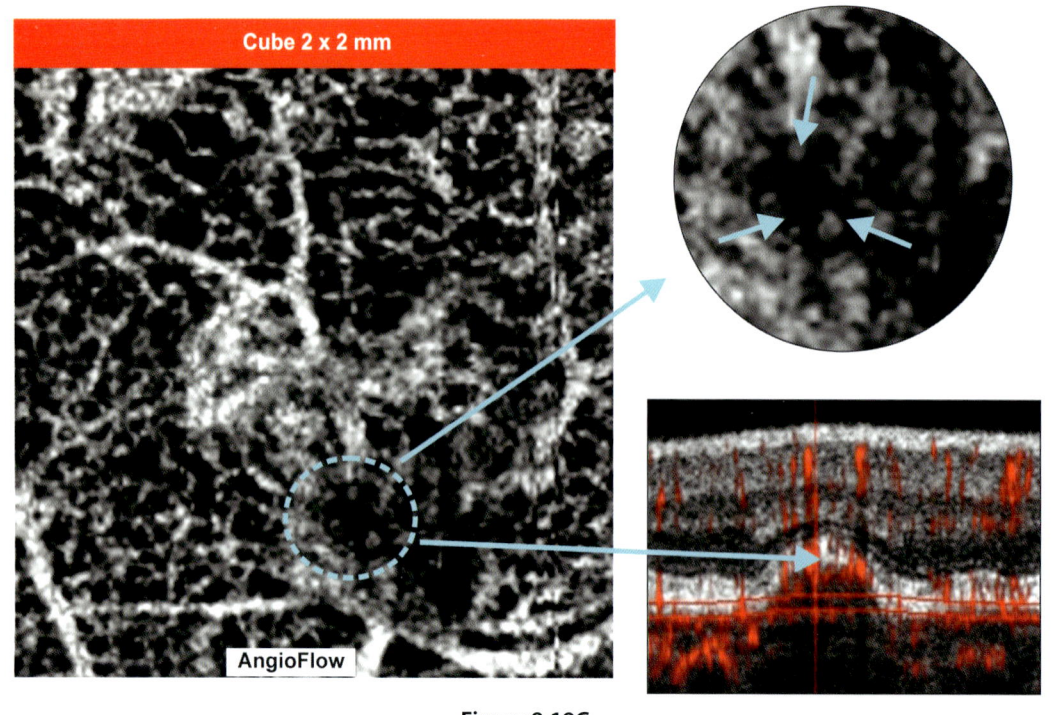

Figure 9.19G

Figures 9.19A to G (A and B) ICGA shows a hypercyanescent branching network and polypoidal dilations; (C) OCTA (Cube 3 × 3 mm) with a slab focused on choriocapillaris shows the branching network with an inhomogeneous decorrelation signal. This latter aspect is probably due to the lack of exudation and the more well-defined borders of the polypoidal lesion; (D) B-scan OCT depitches a little, well-defined PED corresponding to the polyp, and a slightly elevated RPE where the interconnecting network is localized; (E) Cube 3 × 3 mm Angio-OCT with a slab focused on the choriocapillaris visualizes a hyporeflective spot corresponding to the PED, but the polypoidal lesion itself cannot be detected; (F) OCTA with Cube 3 × 3 mm with a slab proportional to PED shows very fine polypoidal dilations corresponding to a slight decorrelation signal; (G) Cube 2 × 2 mm Angio-OCT with a slab focused on the choriocapillaris and proportional to the lesion size succeeds to visualize a mild flow in the polypoidal lesions. Polyps appear as glomerular, interconnected structures

both, the branching network with a slab at the choriocapillary level, as well as the polypoidal dilations with a slab of proportional thickness at the point of RPE detachment containing the polyps.

In this chapter, we will present the characteristics of this disorder on OCT angiography with emphasis on the idiopathic forms of PCV **(Figs 9.15 to 9.19)**.

10
Other Types of Choroidal Neovascularization not Linked to Age-related Macular Degeneration

Leonardo Mastropasqua, Luca Di Antonio

Choroidal neovascularization (CNV) is the leading cause of loss of vision[1] and is mainly associated with age-related macular degeneration (AMD). However, there are other retinal diseases that could be complicated by CNV, affecting the choroid and damaging the retinal pigmented epithelium (RPE) and Bruch's membrane. All these types of CNV share features with AMD.

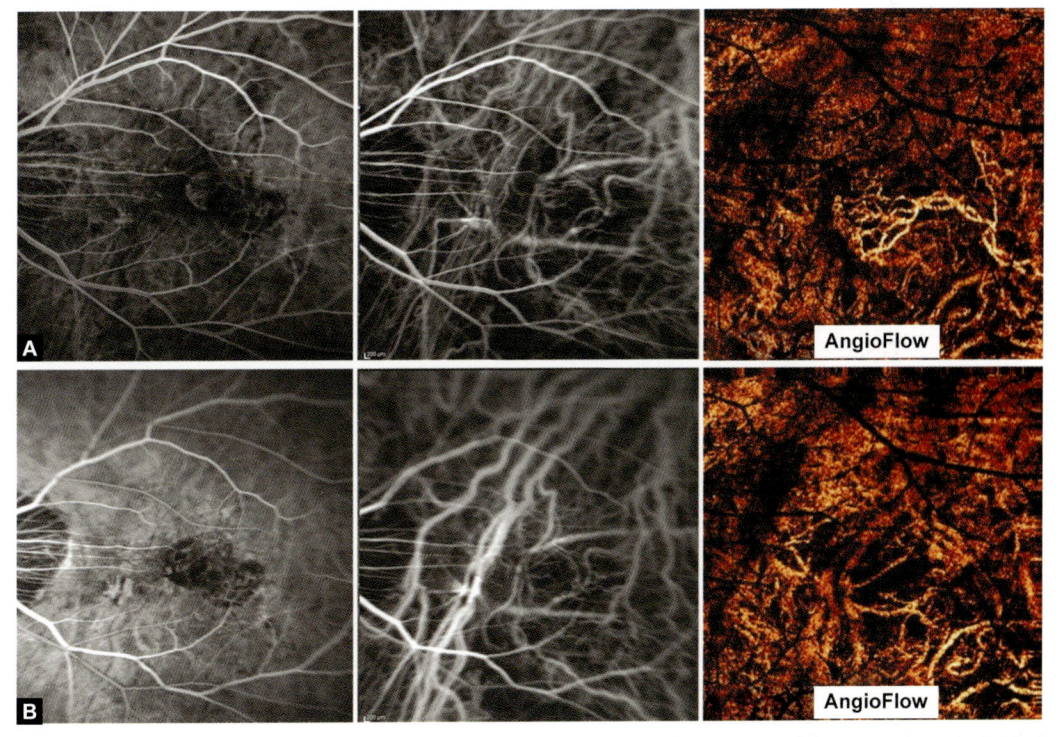

Figures 10.1A and B Multimodal retinal and choroidal imaging of a 56-year-old man with pathological myopia. FA, ICGA and color-mode OCT-A showing neovascular network of mCNV at baseline: (A) OCT-A highlighting the neovascular complex as a high flow of new vessels. FA, ICGA and color-mode OCT-A showing disappearance of choroidal new vessels one month after intravitreal administration of anti-VEGF (B)

88 | Practical Handbook of OCT Angiography

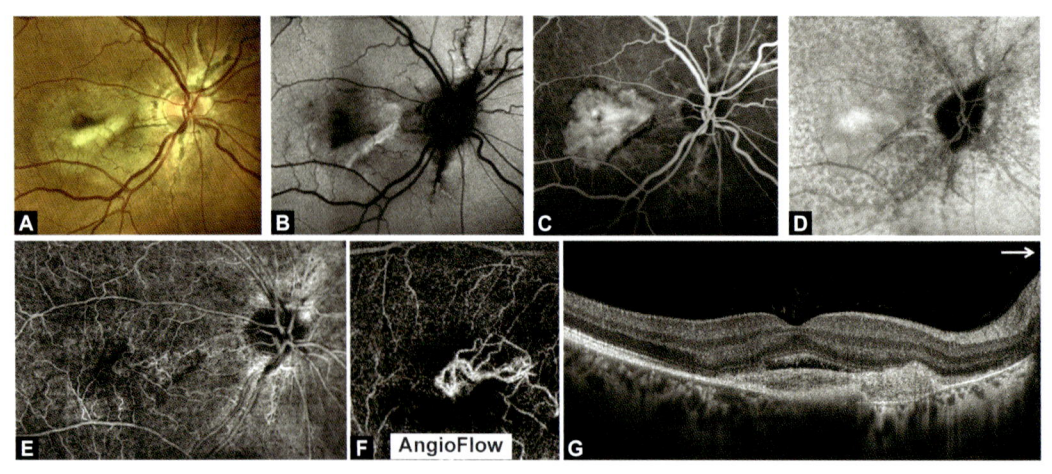

Figures 10.2A to G Multimodal retinal imaging of a 43-year-old man with intermediate β-thalassemia: (A) Color picture showing angioid streaks radiating from optic disc, a yellow-white plaque surrounded by multiple hemorrhages, and vascular tortuosity; (B) Fundus autofluorescence (FAF) showing angioid streaks as ragged dark lines with a variable focal increased FAF along the margins; (C) FA showing angioid streaks as hyperfluorescent lines, and increased hyperfluorescence for staining and pooling of dye (CNV); (D) ICGA depicting a typical "peau d'orange" pattern as hypofluorescent spots and hypofluorescent ragged lines; (E) OCT-A (composition map of 2 partially overlapping 6 × 6 mm scans) highlighting peripapillary angioid streaks and the presence of subfoveal CNV; (F) OCT-A (3 × 3 mm) depicting a "sea-fan" net of abnormal vessels better than standard FA; (G) B-scan showing high-reflective material above RPE and the presence of subretinal fluid

The CNV can occurs as a consequence of several ophthalmologic diseases, including pathological myopia[2] **(Figs 10.1A and B)**, angioid streaks[3] **(Figs 10.2A to G)**, adult onset foveomacular vitelliform dystrophy[4] **(Figs 10.3A to E)**, central serous chorioretinopathy[5] **(Figs 10.4A to F)**, macular telangiectasia[6] **(Figs 10.5A to G)**, polypoidal vasculopathy[7] **(Figs 10.6A to F)** and retinal angiomatous proliferation[8] **(Figs 10.7A to D)**. Early diagnosis is crucial for initiating and guiding the best treatment as a means of preventing progressive and irreversible loss of vision.

Fluorescein angiography (FA), indocyanine green angiography (ICGA) and optical coherence tomography (OCT) are essential tools for the diagnosis and the choice of treatment for CNV. OCT angiography (OCT-A), a novel dye-less method for imaging the retinal and choroidal microvasculature, has been recently introduced into clinical practice.[9]

In this chapter, we highlight the multimodal diagnostic approach to other types of CNV, not linked to AMD, with emphasis on OCT-A findings, especially the ones not obvious with other common gold standard retinal imaging methods.

Other Types of Choroidal Neovascularization not Linked to Age-related Macular Degeneration | **89**

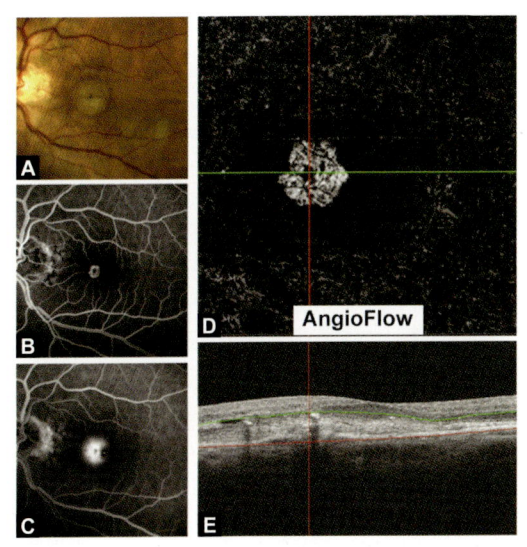

Figures 10.3A to E Multimodal retinal imaging of a 62-year-old woman with vitelliform lesion complicated by type 2 choroidal neovascularization (CNV). Color picture showing yellowish round lesion (A) FA showing early hyperfluorescence (B) and late pooling and leakage of dye (C) OCT angiogram (3 × 3 mm) enhancing a "cartwhell" type 2 CNV (D) B-scan showing reference plane at the level of outer retina (E)

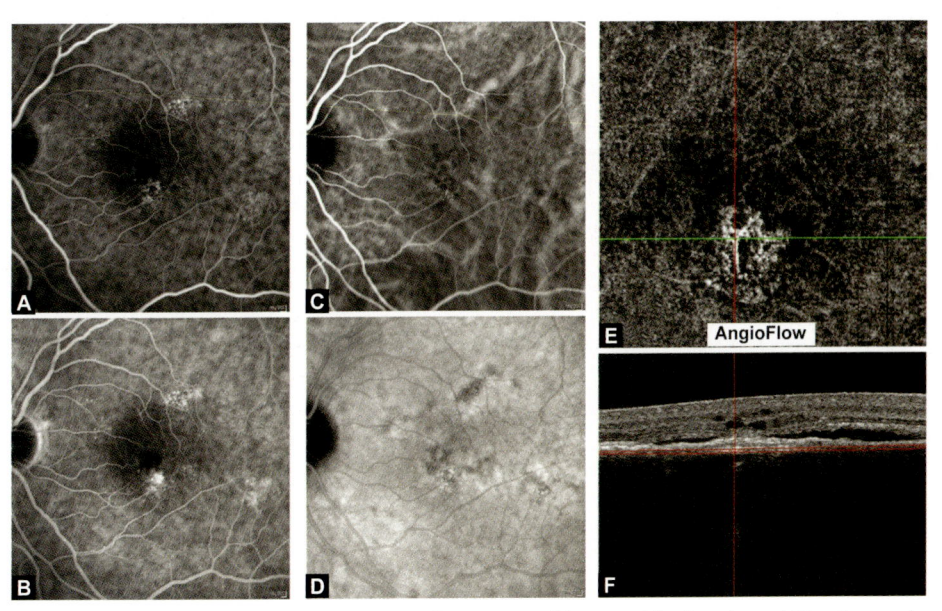

Figures 10.4A to F Multimodal retinal imaging of a 62-year-old man with chronic multifocal central serous chorioretinopathy (CSC) complicated by type 1 choroidal neovascularization (CNV). Early phase of FA showing multiple granular hyperfluorescences (A) Late phase showing a juxtafoveal area of late unusual leakage (B) ICGA showing multiple islands of hyperfluorescence due to choriocapillary hyperpermeability in the early phase (C) Late phase showing wash-out of choroidal islands (D) OCT-A revealing a "tangled" type 2 CNV (E) corresponding B-scan showing the presence of intraretinal cysts, subretinal fluid, and flat pigment epithelium detachment (F)

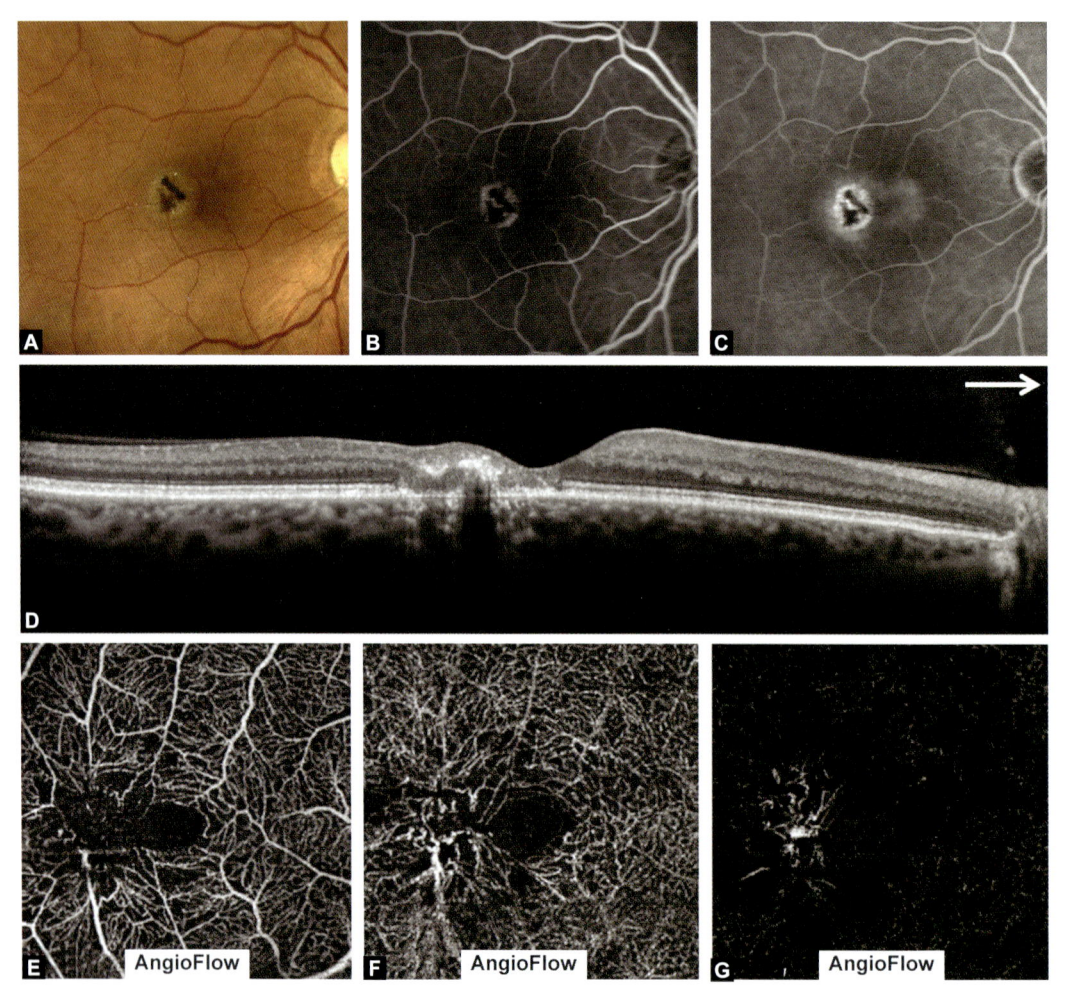

Figures 10.5A to G Multimodal retinal imaging of a 49-year-old woman with proliferative type 2 macular telangiectasia. Color picture showing microvascular abnormalities, crystalline deposits and hyperpigmentation (A). Early phase of FA showing juxtafoveal hyperfluorescence (B). Late phase of FA showing increased hyperfluorescence and leakage (C). Cross-sectional SD-OCT showing retinal thinning, intraretinal hyper-reflectivity and alteration of outer retinal layers (D). OCT-Angiography demonstrating FAZ enlargement and telangiectatic microvascular abnormalities such as right-angled retinal vessels and microaneurysms in the superficial vascular layer (E) and multiple microvascular abnormalities as rarefaction of vascular texture with increase of the intervascular spaces and anastomoses in the perifoveal region of deep vascular layer (F). Note the presence of CNV as a high flow of new vessels into the outer retina (G).

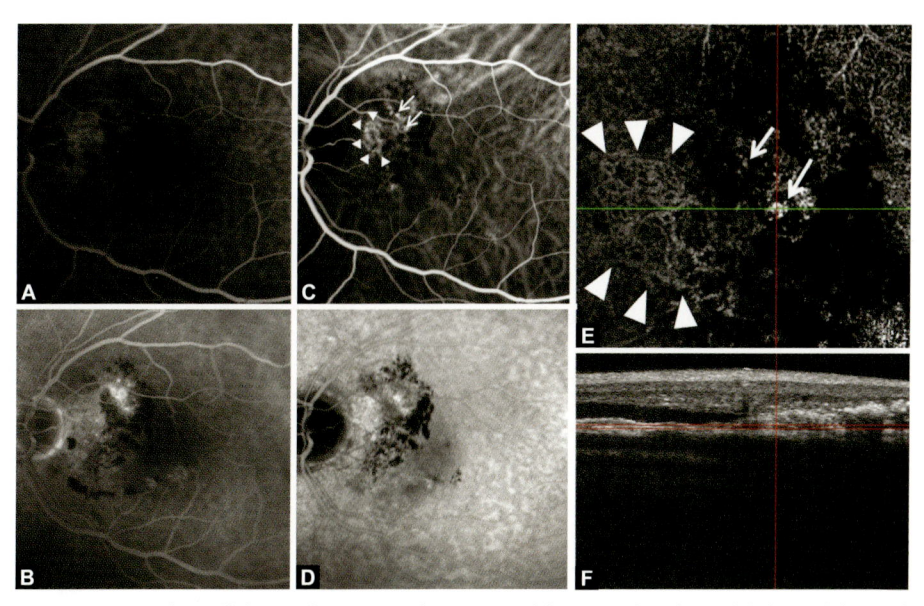

Figures 10.6A to F Multimodal retinal imaging of a 68-year-old man with polypoidal choroidal vasculopathy (PCV). Early phase of FA showing hypofluorescences due to hemorrhages and exudates, and a peripapillary area of increased hyperfluorescence (A) Late phase of angiogram showing pooling and leakage of dye (B) ICGA showing peripapillary branching vascular network (arrowheads) and multiple hyperfluorescent spots due to polyps (white arrows) in the early phase (C) Late phase of ICGA showing washout of the polypoidal lesions (D) OCT-A revealing detailed branching vascular network (arrowheads) and multiple polypoidal lesions (white arrows) (E) B-scan segmented at the level of choriocapillaris showing subretinal fluid, exudates, and polyps below pigment epithelium detachment (F)

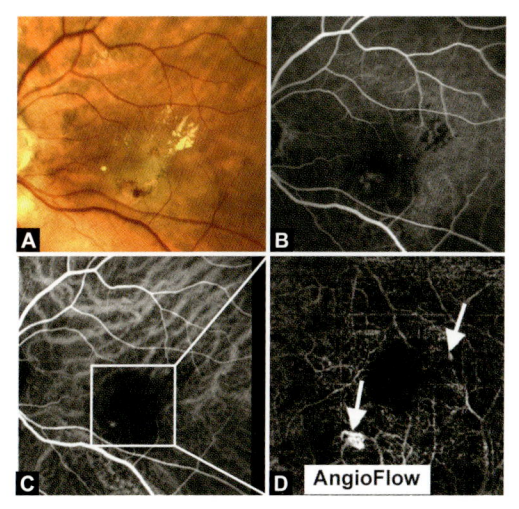

Figures 10.7A to D Multimodal retinal imaging of a 78-year-old woman with double retinal angiomatous proliferations (RAP). Color picture showing hemorrhages and lipid exudation (A). Early FA (B) and ICGA with 3 × 3 mm area boxed off (C) of a 3 × 3 mm OCT-A (D) showing a round RAP lesions (white arrows). A feeding artery and draining venule were noted in both ICGA and OCT-A images

REFERENCES

1. Klein R, Klein BE, Linton KL. Prevalence of age-related maculopathy. The Beaver Dam Eye Study. Ophthalmology. 1992;99:933-43.
2. Wong TY, Ohno-Matsui K, Leveziel N, Holz FG, Lai TY, Gon Yu H, et al. Myopic choroidal neovascularisation: current concepts and update on clinical management. Br J Ophthalmol; 2014. pp.1-8.
3. Barteselli G, Dell'Arti L, Finger RP, Charbel Issa P, Marcon A, Vezzola D, et al. The Spectrum of Ocular Alterations in Patients with b-Thalassemia Syndromes Suggests a Pathology Similar to Pseudoxanthoma Elasticum. Ophthalmology. 2014;121:709-18.
4. Querques G, Regenbogen M, Quijano C, Delphin N, Soubrane G, Souied EH. High-definition optical coherence tomography features in vitelliform macular dystrophy. Am J Ophthalmol. 2008;146:501-7.
5. Quaranta-El Maftouhi M, El Maftouhi A, Eandi CM. Chronic Central Serous Chorioretinopathy Imaged by Optical Coherence Tomographic Angiography. Am J Ophthalmol. 2015;160:581-7.
6. Gass JD, Oyakawa RT. Idiopathic juxtafoveal retinal telangiectasis. Arch Ophthalmol. 1982; 100:769-80.
7. Yannuzzi LA, Sorenson J, Spaide RF, Lipson B. Idiopathic polypoidal choroidal vasculopathy (IPCV). Retina. 1990;10:1-8.
8. Freund KB, Ho IV, Barbazetto IA, Koizumi H, Laud K, Ferrara D, et al. Type 3 neovascularization: the expanded spectrum of retinal angiomatous proliferation. Retina. 2008;28:201-11.
9. Carpineto P, Mastropasqua R, Marchini G, Toto L, Di Nicola M, Di Antonio L. Reproducibility and repeatability of foveal avascular zone measurements in healthy subjects by optical coherence tomography angiography. Br J Ophthalmol; 2015.pp.1-9. doi:10.1136/bjophthalmol 2015;307-30.

11

Subretinal Fibrosis Features in Optical Coherence Tomography Angiography

Eric Souied, Alexandra Miere, Oudy Semoun, Eliana Costanzo, Salomon Yves Cohen

Subretinal fibrosis is the consequence of complex tissue repair mechanisms, appearing either during the natural healing process[1] or during antivascular endothelial growth factor (VEGF) treatment.[2] Key players in its development are connective tissue growth factor (CTGF), platelet-activating

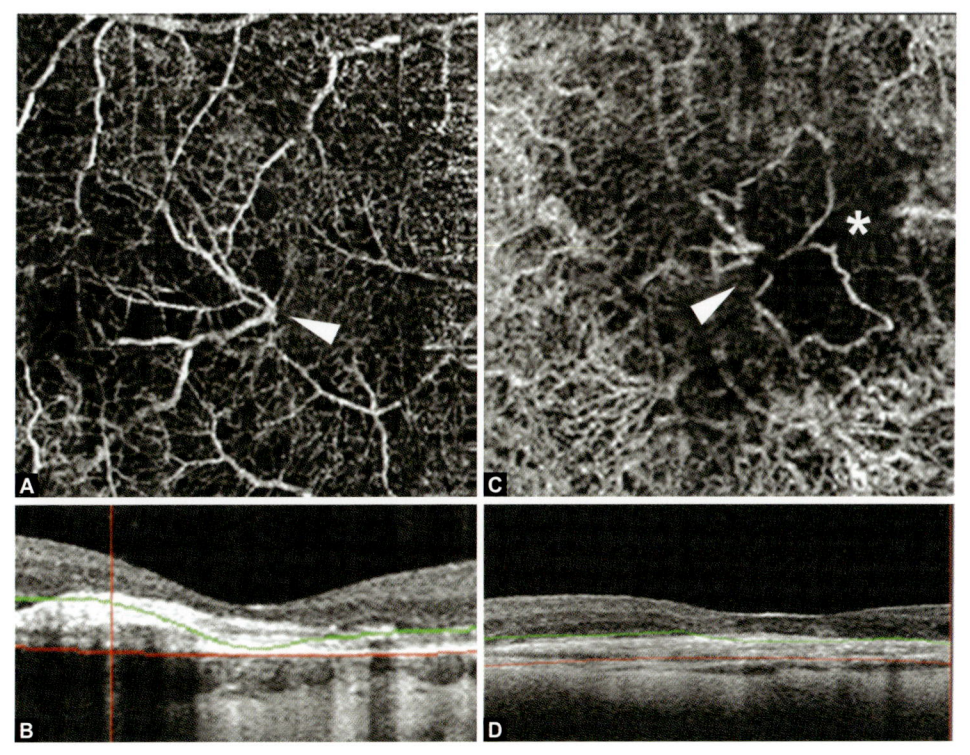

Figures 11.1A to D Optical coherence tomography angiography (OCT-A) of age-related macular degeneration (AMD) patients with subretinal fibrosis with a dead tree neovascular pattern and deep dark area. The OCT-A images in (A) and (C) delineate a vascular network comprising important vessels with high, irregular flow and absence of thinner capillaries (arrowheads). Note the presence of a masking effect generated by the fibrous scar (C) an appearance for which we coined the term deep dark area (asterisk). The corresponding B-scans (B and D) of the OCT-A image in (A and C) show a hyper-reflective subfoveal fibrous scar

94 | Practical Handbook of OCT Angiography

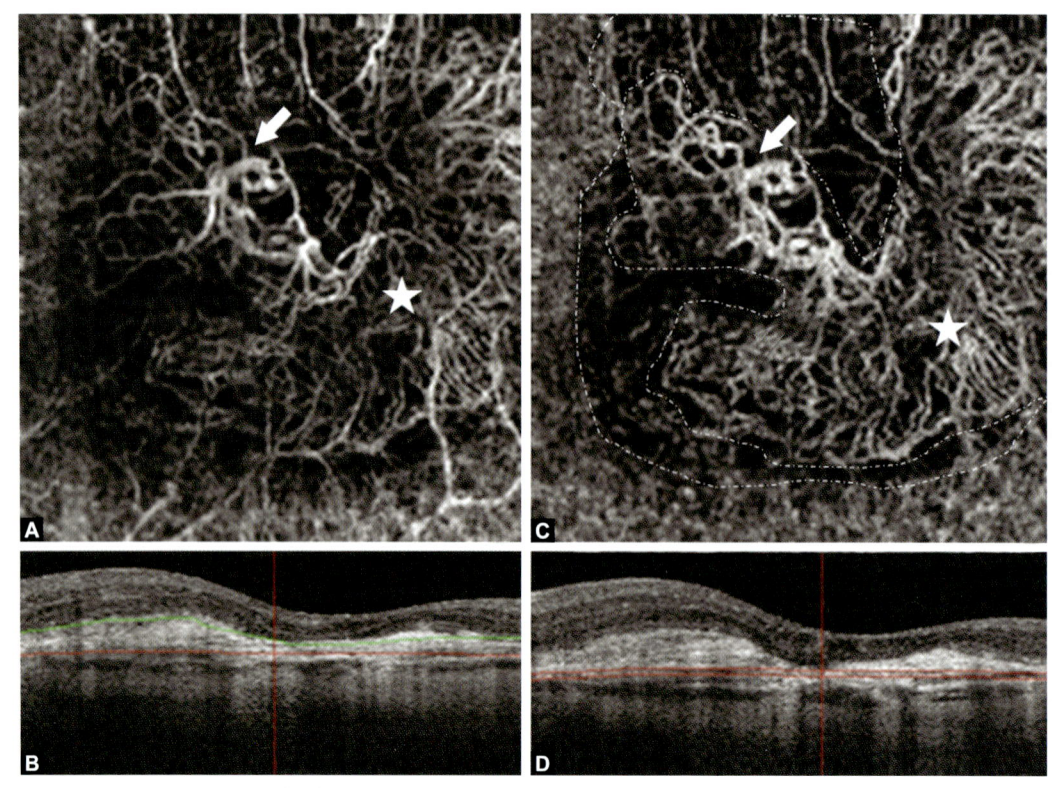

Figures 11.2A to D Optical coherence tomographic angiography (OCT-A) of AMD patients with subretinal fibrosis with tangled network and dark halo features. OCT-A images of the outer retinal segmentation and choriocapillaris segmentation (A and C respectively), and corresponding B-scan (B and D). The tangled neovascular network (white stars) appears as a high-flow structure, comprising thin emerging branches and many collateral branches extending to the surrounding vessels. Vascular loops are visible (arrows), along with a surrounding dark halo (dotted white line), which corresponds to a hypoperfused area (green line) surrounding the choroidal neovascularization

factor (PAF), platelet-activating factor receptor (PAF-R), and macrophage rich peritoneal exudate cells (PEC), as demonstrated by recent studies on animal models.[3-6] With the advent of anti-VEGF therapy and its widespread use in the treatment of exudative age-related macular degeneration (eAMD), there is the possibility of treated choroidal neovascularization (CNV) evolving to result in macular atrophy and/or subretinal fibrosis, both conditions being associated with poor visual outcomes.[7,8]

Subretinal fibrosis is characterized by a well-demarcated, elevated mound of yellowish tissue on fundus examination. This is demonstrated by dye staining in the late frames on fluorescein angiography (FA).[7,8] On spectral domain optical coherence tomography (SD-OCT) fibrosis is identified by the appearance of compact, subretinal hyper-reflective thick lesions, with a possible loss of adjacent retinal pigment epithelium (RPE) and the ellipsoid zone.

Optical coherence tomography angiography (OCT-A) is a depth-resolved imaging technique,[9,10] designed for analysis of retinal and choroidal vessels, which also provides a detailed analysis of the fibrotic scar. OCT-A images of subretinal fibrosis almost constantly reveal a perfused vascular network in addition to collateral architectural changes in the outer retina and the choriocapillaris layer. However, the examination

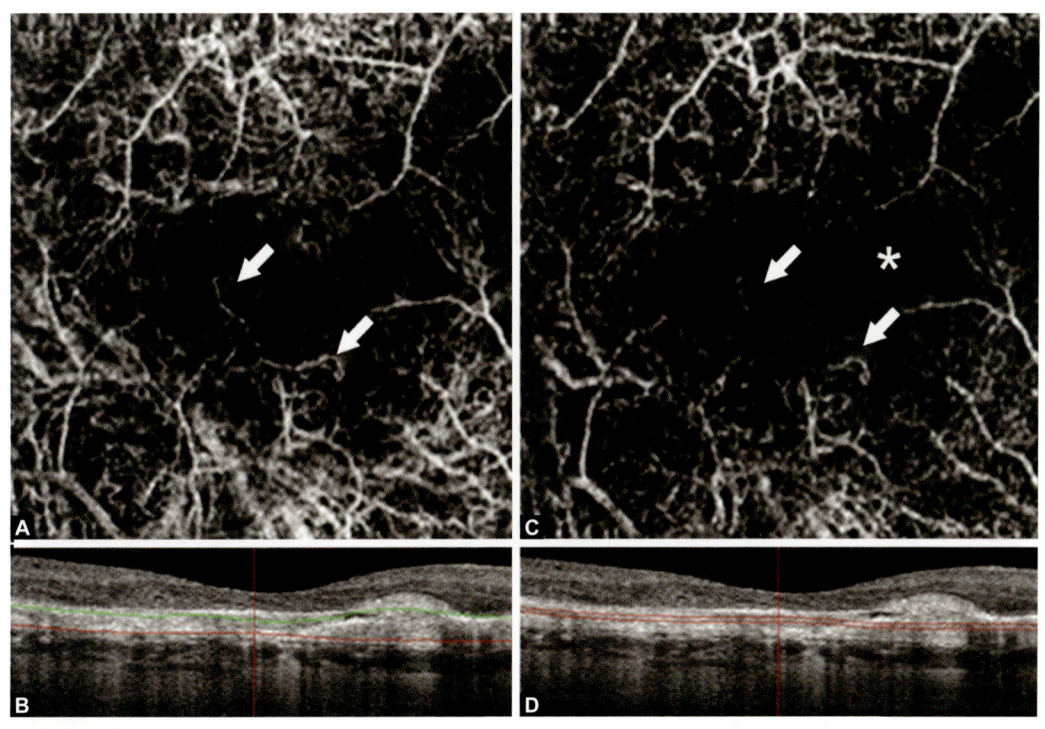

Figures 11.3A to D Optical coherence tomographic angiography (OCT-A) with vascular loop and deep dark area features. OCT-A image of the outer retinal segmentation (A) and corresponding B-scan (B). Two moderately high flow, small vascular loops are visible (arrows). OCT-A image in the choriocapillaris segmentation (C) and corresponding B-scan (D) shows the two vascular loops (arrows) and a black, uniform, deep dark area (asterisk)

may not be interpretable in some of the cases owing to very poor visual acuity, lack of fixation, and lack of patient cooperation.

Three patterns of the neovascular network may be observed inside the fibrotic scar: dead tree, tangled network, and/or vascular loop. *Dead tree pattern* (**Figs 11.1A to D**) is described as a neovascular network consisting of important vessels with irregular flow and absence of thinner capillaries in the segmentation corresponding to the fibrous scar. *Tangled network* (**Figs 11.2A to D**) is characterized by an abnormal high-flow, and interlacing vascular network, which is visible on segmenting the fibrotic scar in OCT-A. Another high flow pattern is vascular loop (**Figs 11.3A to D**), which appears as a convoluted network on OCT-A images. These features of subretinal fibrosis are usually associated with two major phenotypes:

Table 11.1 CNV morphology in vascular fibrosis
Dead tree pattern
Blossoming tree pattern
• Tangled network
• Vascular loop
A dark halo is always present

Abbreviation: CNV, choroidal neovascularization

dead tree or blossoming tree (including tangled network and vascular loop). While the dead tree pattern corresponds to irregular flow in networks formed by major vascular trunks, blossoming tree phenotype is curve-shaped (such as tangled and vascular loop) and correlates with high-flow networks consisting of abundant anastomoses with the adjacent vascularization (**Table 11.1**).

96 | Practical Handbook of OCT Angiography

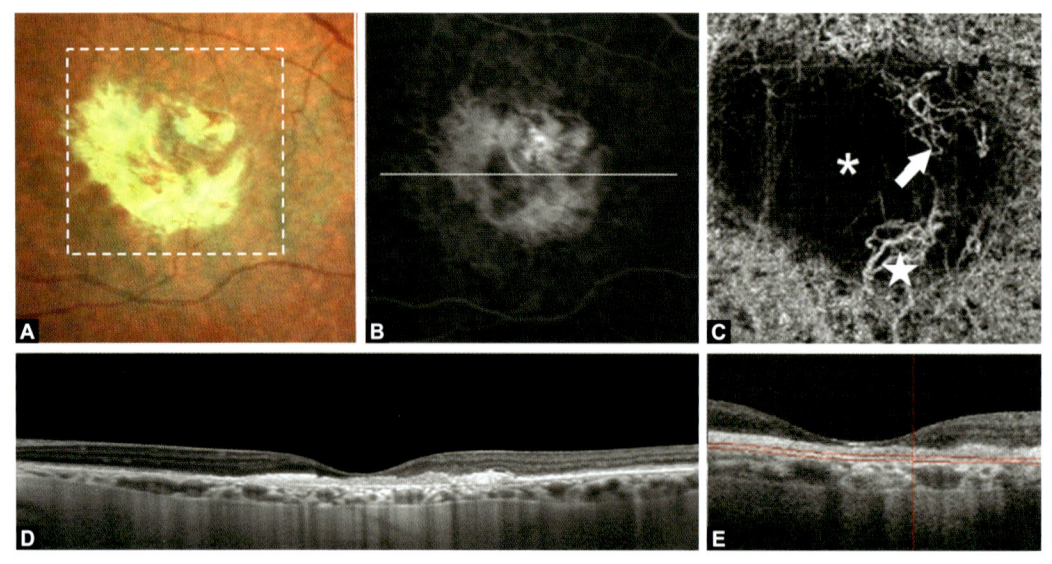

Figures 11.4A to E Multimodal imaging of a patient with exudative AMD and subretinal fibrosis: (A) Color fundus photography shows a well-demarcated, elevated mound of yellow tissue in the macular area. The white dotted square corresponds to the optical coherence tomography angiography (OCT-A) scanning window; (B) Late fluorescein angiography (FA) frame showing staining of the lesion and no distinct visualization of the neovasculature. The white line on (B) Corresponds to the B-scan on (D); (C) OCT-A image of the fibrous scar in the choriocapillaris segmentation, with corresponding B-scan (E) revealing two high-flow, eccentric lesions with different patterns: vascular loop (arrow) and tangled network (white star). Note the presence of a masking effect generated by the scar: deep dark area (asterisk)

OCT-A analysis also identifies the presence of dark lesions: Large deep dark areas and/or a dark halo. The deep dark area represents the masking effect generated by the fibrous scar, while the dark halo corresponds to an obscure ring surrounding the neovascular network **(Figs 11.4A to E)**.

The focus on OCT-A features of subretinal fibrosis occurring in eyes with neovascular AMD reveals distinctive, abnormal vascular networks corresponding to the fibrotic scar. These features were hitherto impossible to identify on FA or SD-OCT alone. The attempt to qualitatively classify these networks observed on OCT-A is of particular interest, both from a clinical and pathophysiological point of view.

REFERENCES

1. Kumar V, Abbas AK, Nelson F. Robbins and Cotran pathologic basis of disease, 9th edn. Philadelphia: Elsevier Saunders; 2014.
2. Hwang JC, Del Priore LV, Freund KB, et al. Development of subretinal fibrosis after anti-VEGF treatment in neovascular age-related macular degeneration. Ophthalmic Surg Lasers Imaging. 2011;42:6-11.
3. Moussad EE, Brigstock DR. Connective tissue growth factor. What's in a name? Mol. Genet. Metab. 2000;71:276-92.
4. Zhang H, Yang Y, Takeda A, et al. A novel platelet-activating factor receptor antagonist inhibits choroidal neovascularization and subretinal fibrosis. PLoS One. 2013;27:8:e68173.
5. Jo YJ, Sonoda KH, Oshima Y, et al. Establishment of a new animal model of focal subretinal fibrosis that resembles disciform lesion in advanced age-related macular degeneration. Invest Ophthalmol Vis Sci. 2011;52:6089-95.
6. Cui W, Zhang H, Liu ZL. Interleukin-6 receptor blockade suppresses subretinal fibrosis in a mouse model. Int J Ophthalmol. 2014;7:194-7.
7. Bloch SB, Lund-Andersen H, Sander B, Larsen M. Subfoveal fibrosis in eyes with neovascular

age-related macular degeneration treated with intravitreal ranibizumab. Am J Ophthalmol. 2013;156:116-24.
8. Channa R, Sophie R, Bagheri S, et al. Regression of choroidal neovascularization results in macular atrophy in anti-vascular endothelial growth factor-treated eyes. Am J Ophthalmol 2015;159: 9-19.
9. Jia Yl, Tan O, Tokayer J, et al. Split-spectrum amplitude-decorrelation angiography with optical coherence tomography. Opt Express. 2012;20:4710-25.
10. Jia Yl, Bailey ST, Wilson DJ, et al. Quantitative optical coherence tomography angiography of choroidal neovascularization in age-related macular degeneration. Ophthalmology 2014; 121:1435-44.

12

Evolution in Time of Flows after Treatment

Bruno Lumbroso, Marco Rispoli

Optical coherence tomography (OCT) angiography allows the observation of new vessels without the blurring caused by fluorescein leakage and has made it easier to understand and follow the evolution of new vessels after treatment.

EARLY CHANGES AFTER TREATMENT

24 Hours after Injection: Marked Regression of the New Vessels

In cases of neovascular membranes treated with anti-VEGF, 24 hours after the injection the vascular network appears smaller and abruptly reduced. The loops are decreased in number, and more importantly, the changes in flow after treatment offer a *fragmented* aspect of the network. The appearance is disrupted and it is difficult to follow the course of the flows. The thinner branches disappear and only the larger vessels coming directly from a feeder vessel or from a bundle of feeder vessels survive. The secondary branches and most of the loops disappear immediately after the intravitreal injection. It is not known if this is due to a slowdown in the flow that makes the capillaries invisible, due to a pulsated flow, which also makes circulation invisible, or owing to a true temporary closure of the involved capillaries. The feeder trunk or a bundle of central branches remain visible.

7–15 Days after the Injection: The Regression of the New Vessels Continues

The decrease in capillary vessels continues until the 10–15th day. In fact, in the two or three days following the injection the capillaries continue to decrease and to disappear markedly, and this decrease continues at a slower pace (**Figs 12.1 to 12.3**).

20–25 Days after the Injection: Progressive Reappearance of the New Vessels

Towards the 20th day, some larger vessels progressively reappear. Only a few branches reappear that seem to be thicker and with a higher flow than seen in the vessels before treatment.

It is not known if this is due to the acceleration of the flow that makes the capillaries visible or due to the effective reopening of the capillaries involved. The density of the small capillaries and of the loops at this stage is appreciably less. The vessels that reappear are less tortuous, and remarkably straighter and thicker.

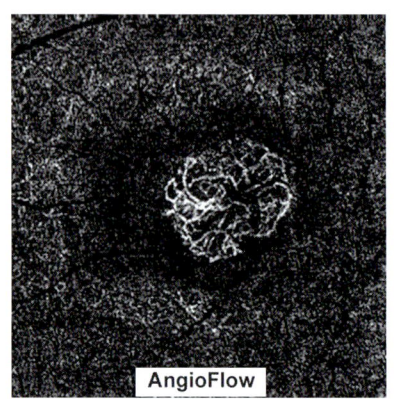

Figure 12.1 Baseline before the injection

Evolution in Time of Flows after Treatment | 99

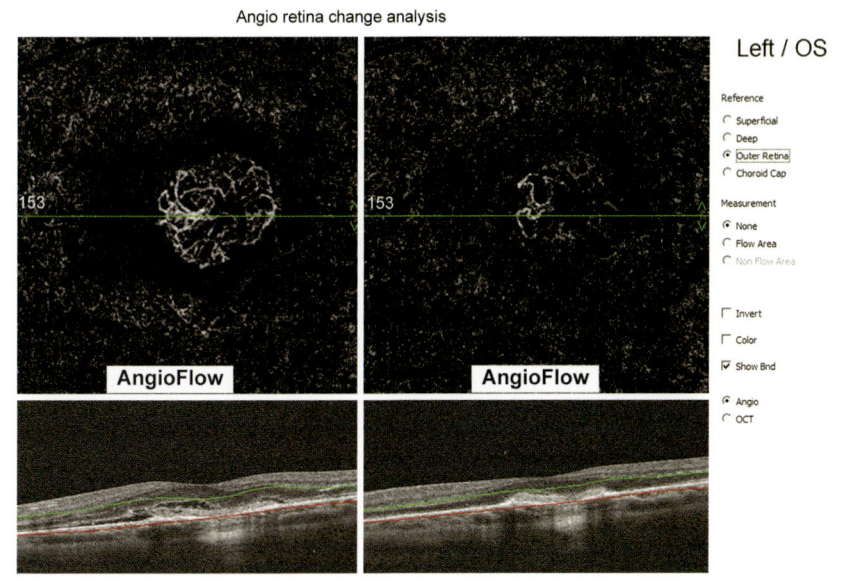

Figure 12.2 24 hours after the injection: regression of new vessels. The network appears to be smaller and abruptly reduced. The loops are less numerous and smaller, and the changes in flow give a *fragmented* disrupted appearance. Thinner branches disappear, while larger vessels coming from the feeder vessel or from the bundle of feeder vessels survive. Secondary branches are less visible

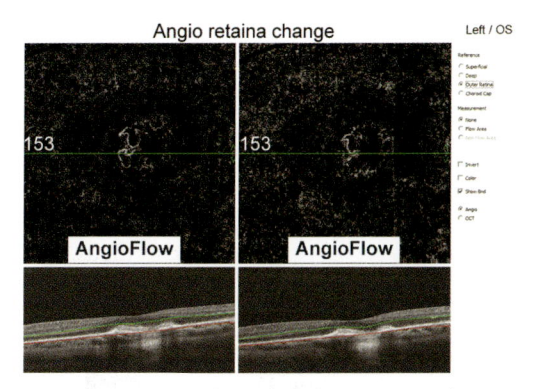

Figure 12.3 7–15 days after the injection: the new vessels continue to regress. The decrease in capillary density continues and progresses until day 10/15. The capillaries continue to decrease and disappear

3 or 4 Weeks after the Injection: Further Reappearance of Larger New Vessels

After 3 or 4 weeks, the main vessels reappear, which in general, follow the course of the original vessels but are thicker, less winding and have a faster flow. The increase in flow modifies the walls and leads to histological changes, especially vessel arterialization.

The new vessels that reappear after treatment are generally wider and thicker compared to the naive vessels. They have an increased flow and look *arterialized*, but globally, their surface is smaller. Some correspond to the vessels that had disappeared, especially to the ones that disappeared most recently. Others are new branches or pre-existing thin branches whose diameter increases, and course becomes less tortuous and more obvious. Spaide compares them to bonsai trees where repeated pruning and thinning out of the smaller branches leads to an enlargement of the trunk.

After 40–50 Days: The Neovascular Membrane is Visible Again

In the first recurrence, the surface of the neovascular membrane is smaller and different in appearance, with lesser thin branches, lesser loops and the presence of a vascular network of fewer, thicker and straighter vessels.

Subsequent treatments lead to further increases in flow, increases in trunk diameter and greater arterialization. The overall surface of the neovascular membrane is generally smaller and has a different appearance compared to that of the naive membrane, with less branches, less loops, and a simpler and less dense network of thicker and straighter vessels **(Figs 12.4 to 12.6)**.

Long-term Evolution Over the Years after Many Injections

Spaide described the appearance of the new vessels and of the fibrous scar after following fairly long evolutions after treatment (50 or more injections of anti-VEGF). A perfused neovascular network persists, formed by arterialized vessels that are less winding and more rigid. Inside the fibrous scar it is possible to observe some large vessels with an irregular flow; thin capillaries or fine loops are not visible while vessels with a large diameter and high flow can be seen. Spaide compares this evolution to the creation of a bonsai tree, where the repeated pruning of the small branches increases the size of the trunk.

Long-term Evolution of the Fibrous Scar

Spaide describes the fibrous scar that contains the residual vascular network (see Chapter 11) **(Figs 12.7 and 12.8)**. The OCT images highlight a perfused neovascular network in the subretinal fibrosis. According to Spaide, inside the fibrous scar, three neovascular patterns can be seen, which he calls the "dead tree" pattern, the "tangled network" pattern and a "vascular loop" pattern. The remaining new vessels form large patterns with irregular flow, which, in general, have no capillary structure but only large vessels. In some other cases, the high-flow vessels have the appearance of a thick network of tangled loops of new vessels.

OCT angiography also makes it possible to evaluate the presence of a dark round shadow behind and around the neovascular network.

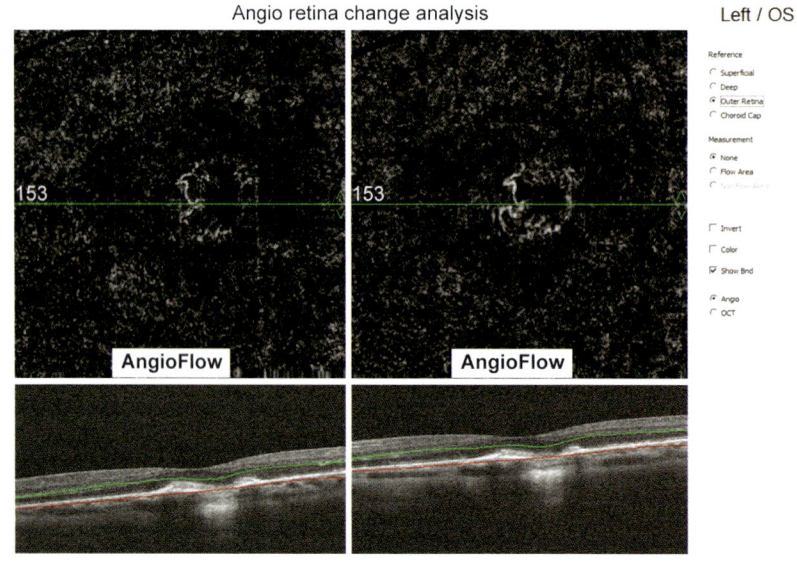

Figure 12.4 20–25 days after the injection: progressive reappearance of the new vessels. Towards the twentieth day, some larger vessels progressively reappear. Only a few branches reappear, and they are thicker and have a higher flow than in the vessels prior to treatment. The vessels that reappear are less winding, straighter and thicker

Evolution in Time of Flows after Treatment | **101**

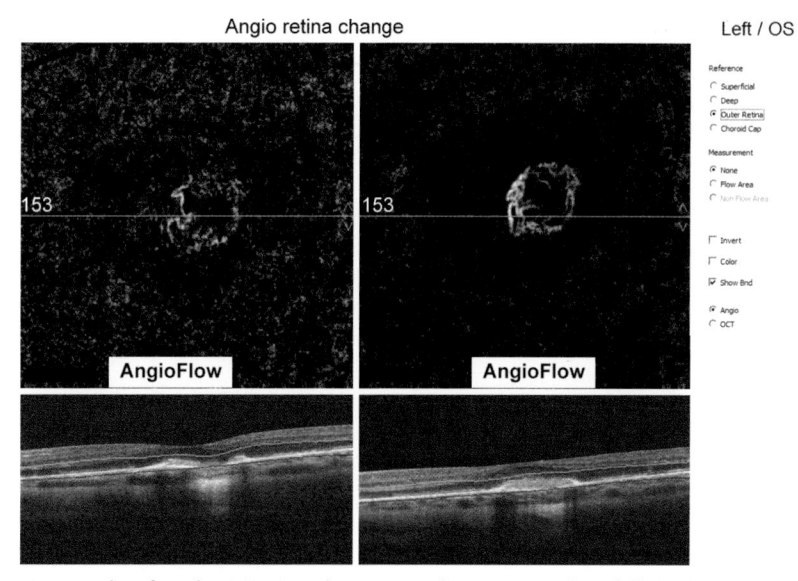

Figure 12.5 3–4 weeks after the injection: larger vessels reappear. They follow the course of the original vessels but are now thicker and less winding, with a higherflow. The increase in flow and reflects on the vessel walls leading to vessel arterialization. The new vessels that form again are, in general wider and thicker, compared to the naive vessels. They show an increased flow, and appear *arterialized* but globally their surface is smaller. Some seem to correspond to the vessels that had disappeared, especially the ones that disappeared more recently. There are new vascular branches or pre-existing thin branches whose diameter increased; they are less winding, straighter and more evident. Spaide compares them to bonsai trees where repeated pruning and thinning of the smaller branches leads to an enlargement of the trunk

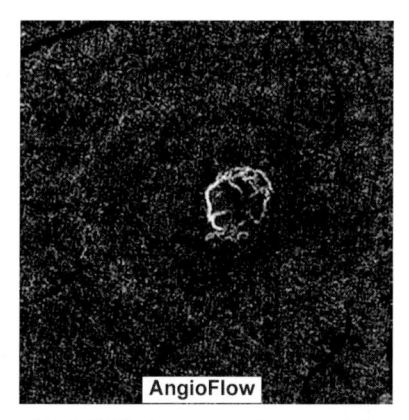

Figure 12.6 CNV shows san increased flow, and appears arterialized with smaller surface. Most branches are increased in diameter, they are less winding, straighter and more evident

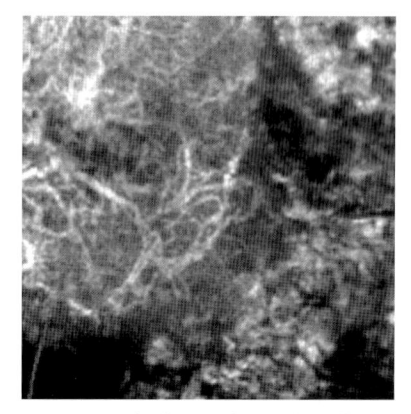

Figure 12.7 Residual vessels inside a fibrous scar: it is possible to observe some large vessels with an irregular flow; no thin capillaries or fine loops are visible while vessels with a large diameter and high flow can be seen

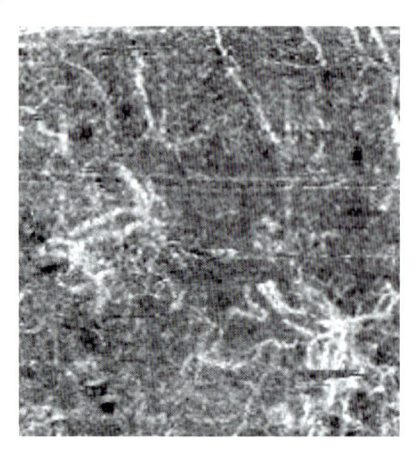

Figure 12.8 Residual vessels inside a fibrous scar: large vessels with irregular flow. Spaide compares this evolution to the creation of a bonsai tree, where the repeated pruning of the small branches increases the size of the trunk

BIBLIOGRAPHY

1. Kuehlewein L, Sadda SR, Sarraf D. OCT angiography and sequential quantitative analysis of type 2 neovascularization after ranibizumab therapy. Eye (Lond). 2015;29(7):932-5.
2. Lumbroso B, Rispoli M, Savastano MC. Longitudinal optical coherence tomography-angiography study of type 2 naive choroidal neovascularization early response after treatment. Retina. 2015;35(11):2242-51.
3. Pechauer AD, Jia Y, Liu L, Gao SS, Jiang C, Huang D. Optical coherence tomography angiography of peripapillary retinal blood flow response to hyperoxia. Invest Ophthalmol Vis Sci. 2015;56(5):3287-91.
4. Spaide RF. Optical coherence tomography angiography signs of vascular abnormalization with antiangiogenic therapy for choroidal neovascularization. Am J Ophthalmol. 2015;160(1):6-16.

13

Optic Nerve and Glaucoma

Michel Puech

Use of optical coherence tomography (OCT) angiography is well described for macular diseases. OCT angiography-based segmentation can provide very useful information for the diagnosis and follow-up of age-related macular degeneration. More recent developments in OCT angiography allow this technology to be applied in the vascular analyses of optic nerve head and peripapillary region.

In current practice, a very dense superficial peripapillary vascular network can be observed with RTVue-XR Avanti (Optovue, Fremont, CA, USA) and split-spectrum amplitude decorrelation angiography (SSADA) software. This vascular network is not clearly seen on fluorescein angiography (FA). Segmentation of OCT angiography can select very superficial images with *en face* OCT focused on the peripapillary area. Accuracy of the OCT angiography system can detect very small blood flows in very small vessels. OCT angiography usually identifies a very dense superficial vascular network, probably mixed with nerve fibers. This superficial vascular network seems to be reduced in patients with glaucoma.

Correlating the density of this vascular network on OCT angiography with other imaging procedures (retinal nerve fiber layer [RNFL], ganglion cell complex [GCC], Visual field) can demonstrate a reliable identification of the stage of the glaucoma.

OPTICAL COHERENCE TOMOGRAPHY ANGIOGRAPHY AROUND THE OPTIC DISC

The OCT angiography can show density variations of this superficial vascular network. Areas with local reduction of vascular density or very large reductions can be easily appreciated. These reductions appear as dark areas. Further, in some patients, the reduction of vascular density network extends all around the optic nerve head (ONH). As this reduction of vascularization was often identified in glaucomatous patients, we analyzed patients referred by ophthalmologist for glaucoma imaging (Visual field, RNFL and GCC). Based on our analyses, OCT angiography identifies three groups of patients.

Group 1: Very dense peripapillary vascular network with no reduction in the vascular network. These patients most often have no reduction in the RNFL or GCC and have a normal visual field **(Fig. 13.1A)**.

Group 2: Localized vascular network reduction with reduction of RNFL, GCC and visual field either involving a very small area, or a larger area **(Fig. 13.1B)**.

Group 3: Extended vascular network reduction involving all quadrants **(Fig. 13.1C)**.

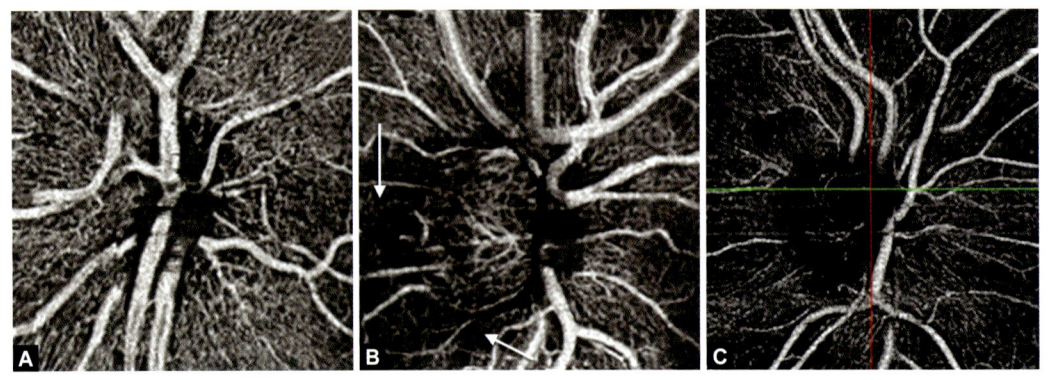

Figures 13.1A to C OCT angiography with analysis of superficial retinal network around the optic disc: (A) Very dense superficial network in case of patients without glaucoma; (B) Localized reduction of superficial vascularization seen as dark areas in the temporal quadrant (arrows); (C) Dark area all around the optic disc in case of advanced glaucoma

Correlation of OCT angiography findings with the glaucoma criteria is observed with respect to changes in RNFL, GCC and visual field. Most often, patients in group 1 have no RNFL, GCC or visual field defects. Group 2 is associated with reduction of RNFL, GCC and visual fields corresponding to reductions in the localized peri-optic vascular network **(Fig. 13.2)**. Group 3 shows large reductions of perioptic vascular network involving all quadrants consistent with extensive glaucoma disease involving RNFL, GCC and visual fields **(Fig. 13.3)**.

These preliminary observations regarding OCT angiography in glaucoma, with evidence of correlation between glaucoma stage and peri-optic vascular network reduction, demonstrate the strong relationship of glaucoma with vascular factors. There is a need for further studies with large series of patients and the application of quantitative approaches, including flow index, vascular density or avascular zone detection, to achieve statistical correlation.

VASCULARIZATION INSIDE THE OPTIC DISC

The OCT angiography with RTVue-XR Avanti (Optovue, Inc.) can demonstrate the vascular network inside the optic nerve head and localize the underlying lamina cribrosa. The changes in the vascular network are similar to the present criteria

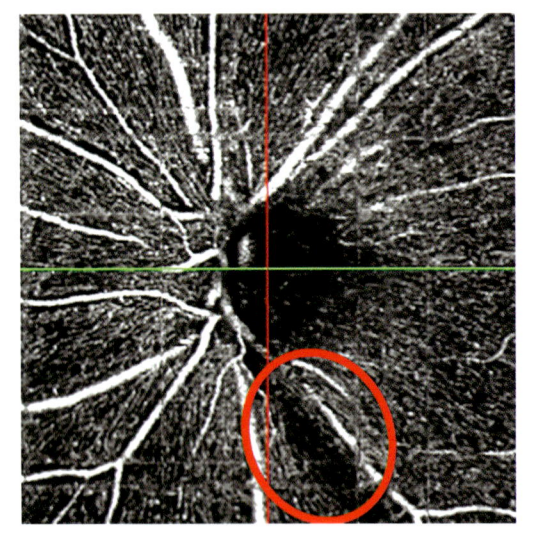

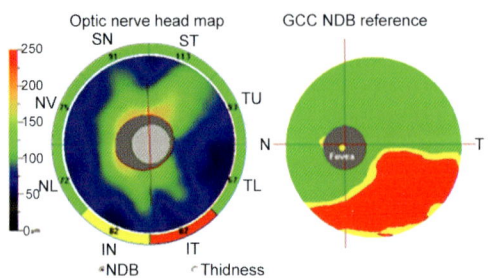

Figure 13.2 Spatial correlation between dark area zone on *en face* OCT angiography map (circle), RNFL and GCC

Optic Nerve and Glaucoma | **105**

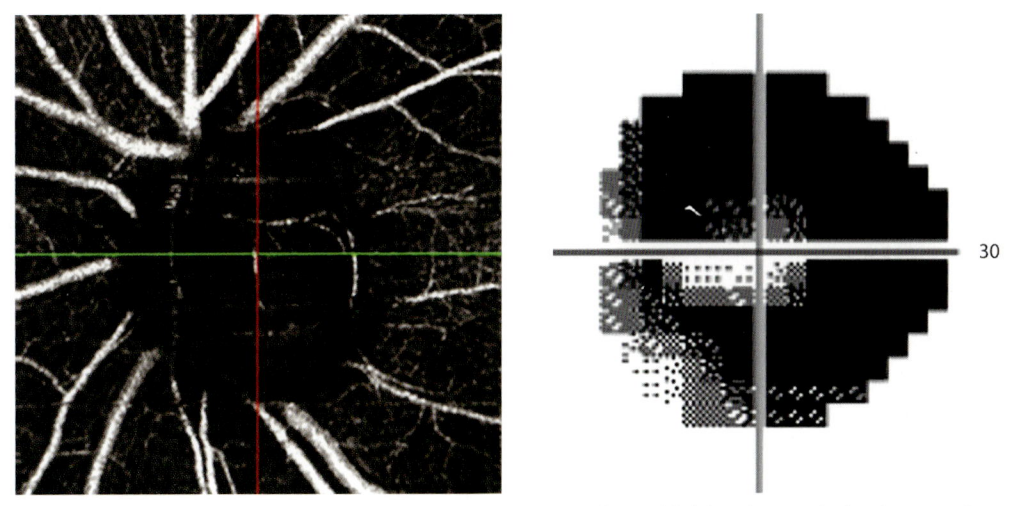

Figure 13.3 Advanced glaucoma with large reduction of visual field and extended reduction of OCT-angiography analysis all around the optic disc

regarding perioptic superficial vascular network: presence of low blood flow and very small diameter vessels. On *en face* OCT angiography, the papillary network and the perioptic disc superficial network are not in the same plane owing to the anatomy of the papilla. We imaged a few optic nerve heads in cases with papillary drusen and demonstrated continuity of the two vascular networks **(Fig. 13.4)**. It is our assumption that vascular network around and within the optic nerve head have a role in the nourishment of optic fibers.

In advanced glaucoma, reduction in the vascular network is similar within and around the optic disc **(Figs 13.5A and B)**. Imaging in these cases can provide a subjective assessment of the vascular network within the optic nerve head. However, the use of quantitative index has a limited accuracy in this context owing to the acquisition artifact related to large retinal vessels.

CONCLUSION

The OCT-angiography is a revolutionary modality for macular imaging and age-related macular degeneration. OCT angiography is a very precise tool to evaluate superficial vascular network in the imaging of the optic nerve head. The correlation

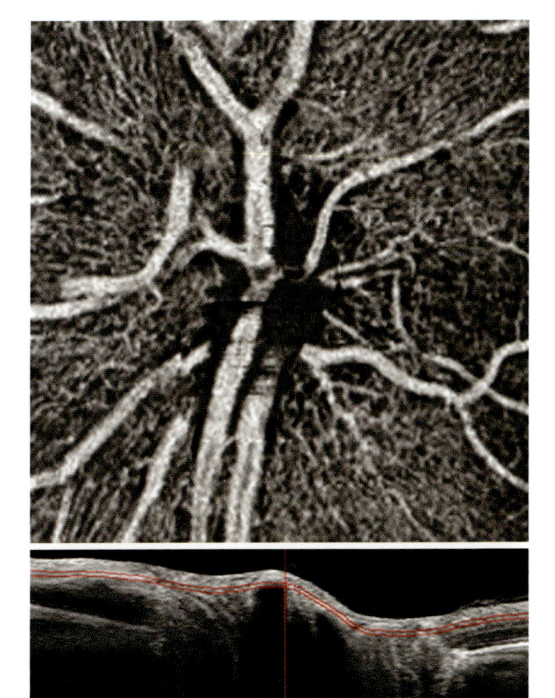

Figure 13.4 OCT-angiography demonstrates a continuous superficial network around and inside the optic disc in a case of optic nerve head drusen

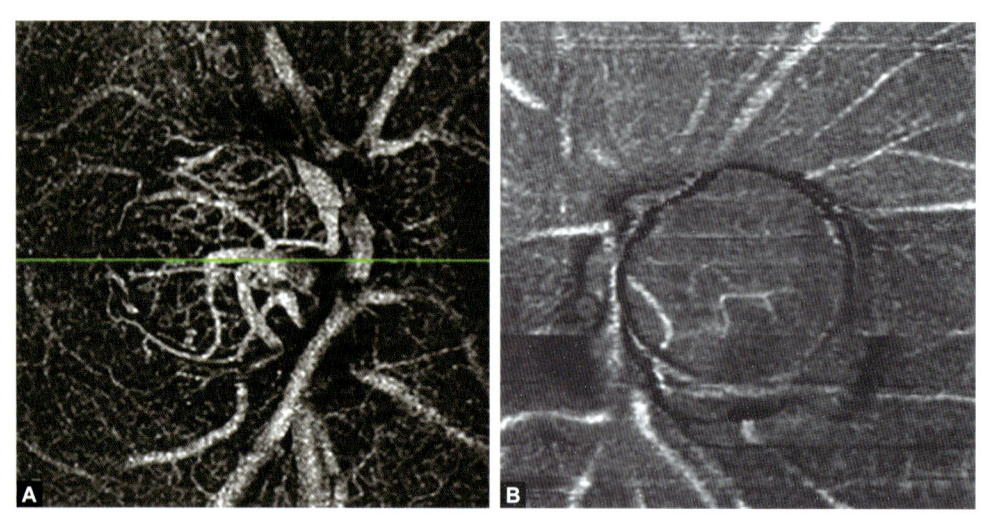

Figures 13.5A and B Superficial vascular layers within the optic disc analyzed by OCT angiography: (A) OCT angiography with a very dense superficial vascular network in a patient without glaucoma; (B) Very dark optic disc appearance in advanced glaucoma

between glaucoma disease and reduction of the superficial vascularization is confirmed by other tests of glaucoma (RNFL, GCC, Visual field). Though the imaging of optic nerve head correlates well with glaucoma, large vessel artefacts limit the use of this system for vascular network analysis. Newer developments in quantitative approaches are needed to include OCT angiography in routine practice for the follow-up of patients with glaucoma.

BIBLIOGRAPHY

1. Baumann B, Potsaid B, Kraus MF, et al. Total retinal blood flow measurement with ultrahigh speed swept source/Fourier domain OCT. Biomed Opt Express. 2011;2(6):1539-52.
2. Huang D, Chopra V, Lu AT, et al. Advanced Imaging for Glaucoma Study-AIGS Group. Does optic nerve head size variation affect circumpapillary retinal nerve fiber layer thickness measurement by optical coherence tomography? Invest Ophthalmol Vis Sci. 2012;53(8):4990-7.
3. Huang D, Puech M, Jia Y, et al. OCT Angiography and Glaucoma, Clinical OCT-Angiography Atlas, Bruno Lumbroso, 2014, Jaypee, Ch 28.
4. Hwang JC, Konduru R, Zhang X, et al. Relationship among visual field, blood flow, and neural structure measurements in glaucoma. Invest Ophthalmol Vis Sci. 2012;53(6):3020-6.
5. Jia Y, Morrison JC, Tokayer J, et al. Quantitative OCT angiography of optic nerve head blood flow. Biomed Opt Express. 2012;3(12):3127-37.
6. Jia Y, Tan O, Tokayer J, et al. Split-spectrum amplitude-decorrelation angiography with optical coherence tomography. Opt Express. 2012;20(4):4710-25.
7. Jia Y, Wei E, Wang X, et al. Optical coherence tomography angiography of optic disc perfusion in glaucoma. Ophthalmology. 2014;121(7):1322-32.
8. Lumbroso B, Huang D, Jia Y, Fujimoto, et al. Optical coherence tomography angiography: New clinical terminology. Clinical guide to Angio-OCT. JAYPEE; 2014. pp. 5-7.
9. Pechauer AD, Jia Y, Liu L, et al. Optical Coherence Tomography Angiography of Peripapillary Retinal Blood Flow Response to Hyperoxia. Invest Ophthalmol Vis Sci. 2015;56(5):3287-91.
10. Sehi M, Goharian I, Konduru R, et al. Retinal blood flow in glaucomatous eyes with single-hemifield damage. Ophthalmology. 2014;121(3):750-8.
11. Tokayer J, Jia Y, Dhalla AH, et al. Blood flow velocity quantification using split-spectrum amplitude-decorrelation angiography with optical coherence tomography. Biomed Opt Express. 2013;4(10):1909-24.
12. Wang X, Jia Y, Spain R, et al. Optical coherence tomography angiography of optic nerve head and parafovea in multiple sclerosis. Br J Ophthalmol. 2014;98(10):1368-73.

14 Comparing Fluorescein Angiography with Optical Coherence Tomography Angiography

Bruno Lumbroso, Marco Rispoli

The recent use of optical coherence tomography (OCT) angiography in routine clinical practice, and its rapid adoption, demand that its characteristics and clinical applications, and above all its usefulness in comparison to fluorescein angiography (FA) be analyzed.

To compare fluorescein angiography and OCT angiography, we applied a logical method based on coherent criteria to decipher the data provided by the two angiography methods. This is not an easy or a simple process. The logical method is divided into two parts: the analysis, which further divides each argument or image into its constituent elements, and the synthesis, which then unites the elements that were isolated. This method results in very practical conclusions.

The general observations can be summarized as follows:

The OCT angiography can provide the exact cast of blood circulation. It can provide precise data regarding intravascular shape, branching of vessels till the smallest capillaries, anastomoses, shunts, and capillary loss, among other details.

We are able to measure and quantify exactly, the blood flow, capillary density, capillary loss and other quantifiable elements. However, it does not provide some information that FA offers us.

Fluorescein angiography (FA) demonstrates damages and deterioration of the vascular walls, that are not yet visible histologically. Wall leakage and wall staining are functional lesions not yet obvious on OCT angiography.

Engineers and physicists will soon provide solutions to quantify wall alterations that at present seem only qualitative.

FLUORESCEIN ANGIOGRAPHY

The FA provides for the diagnosis and follow-up of almost all retinal and sub-retinal disorders. It also aids in deciding the treatment to apply as well as in the assessing the efficacy of the applied treatment.

Side Effects

Fluorescein angiography is an invasive exam associated with discomforting side effects such as nausea, vomiting, and syncope. It is also associated sometimes with severe, though rare, complications like general allergic reactions and Quincke's edema. Severe cardiac and cardiovascular complications are extremely rare but unfortunately there have been cases of anaphylactic shock in one out of a million cases. *In spite of these drawbacks, that at times may be quite severe, fluorescein angiography is the current gold standard* for the study of all retinal vascular disorders.

Angiography with fluorescein provides two-dimensional pictures, hence the vessels appear to be overlaid and superimposed on one another with summation and interference between the various fluorescent images. Another characteristic of traditional fluorescein angiography is that it is a dynamic investigation and hence the images are temporally sequenced as initial, intermediate and late frames. Therefore, the study has a definite beginning and an end.

Repeating an invasive exam is not well accepted by patients or physicians. Often clinicians are hesitant in planning a fluorescein angiography test in elderly people, patients with cardiac conditions and in pregnant women. OCT angiography enables frequent repetition of the examination and thus minimizes the need for an invasive investigation like fluorescein angiography. This noninvasive test is reassuring to both patients and their ophthalmologists as it can be repeated without the need for anesthetists, nurses or dye injections.

Advantages of Fluorescein Angiography

The main advantage of fluorescein angiography is that it demonstrates the leaking of the dye, its pooling in the intraretinal and subretinal cavities and staining of the vascular walls. Fluorescein angiography enables the examination of the retinal periphery beyond the vascular arcades and the vortex veins (**Fig. 14.1**).

OCT Angiography

The OCT Angiography is a three-dimensional examination. The images are extracted from a cube and are, in general, parallel to Bruch's membrane or to the pigment epithelium. OCT angiography is also a static examination, implying that there are no differences between the images at any given time. Even though OCT angiography is based on the movement of the blood, the retinal images are static. As of now, with OCT angiography, the retinal periphery beyond the vascular arcades cannot be examined and the area that can be studied at a time does not exceed 8 mm × 8 mm, though this is expected to increase to areas of 12 mm × 12 mm.

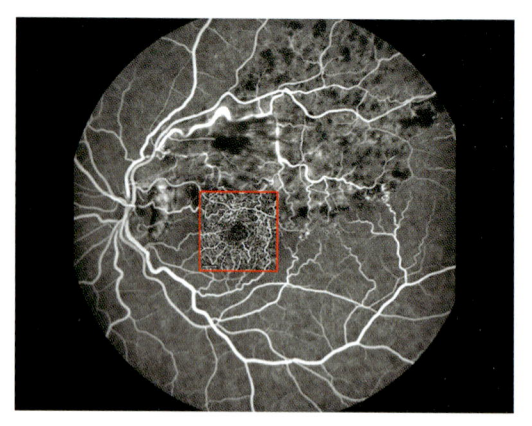

Figure 14.1 Fluorescein angiography of a branch retinal vein occlusion showing that the first 3 × 3 mm OCT angiography covered only a small part of the posterior pole. Optovue AngioVue imaging may now cover all posterior pole with the optic disc

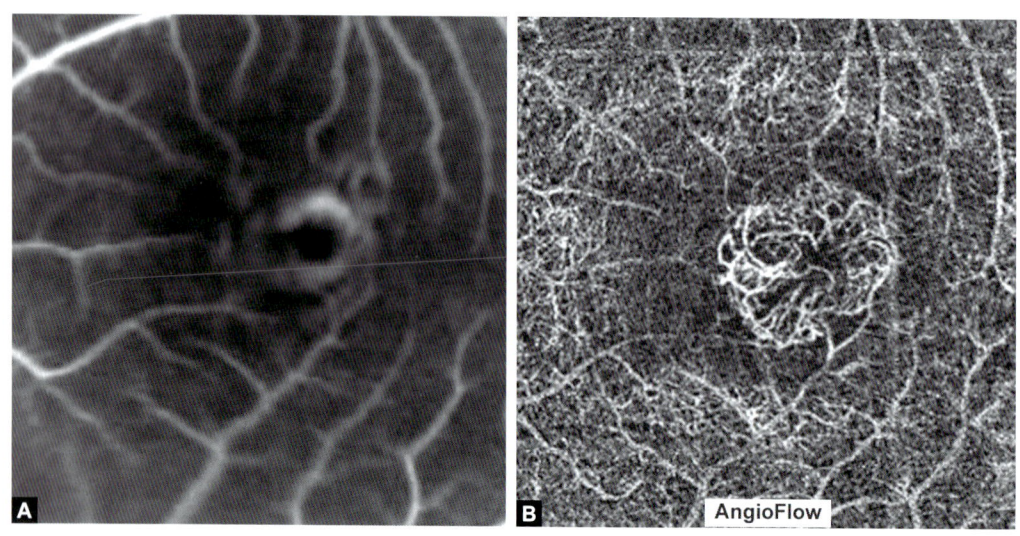

Figures 14.2A and B Fluorescein angiography and OCT angiography of a choroidal neovascularization. Leakage does not allow a good vision of the CNV features when using FA. OCT angiography allows a clear and sharp vision of the small capillaries

Advantages of OCT Angiography

The main advantage of *OCT angiography* is that, unlike fluorescein angiography, it is not hampered by dye leakage or its pooling in the intra and subretinal cavities, and there is no staining of the vessel walls. OCT angiography provides clear images of the vessel morphology of a given layer *without being masked by the influence of staining, pooling and leakage, and window effect as* in fluorescein angiography. OCT angiography enables immediate evaluation of the morphology of fine vessels, without the evaluation being hampered by the diffusion of a cloud of dye **(Figs 14.2 to 14.4)**.

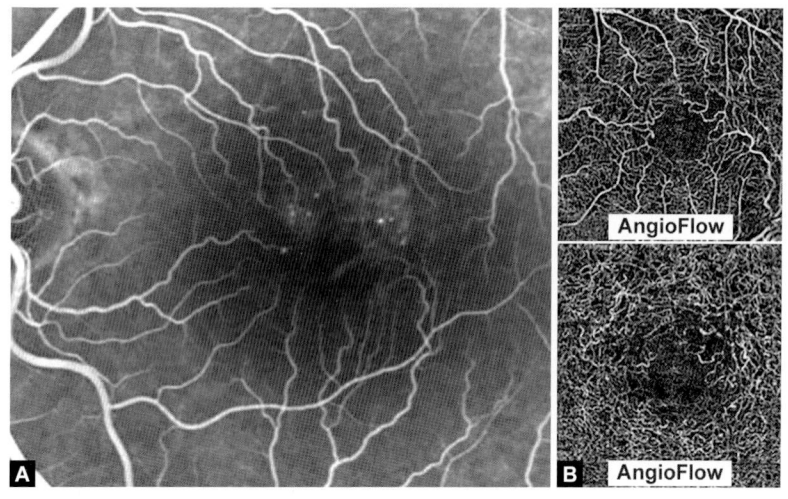

Figures 14.3A and B Fluorescein angiography and OCT angiography of a nonproliferative diabetic retinopathy. Leakage does not allow a good vision of the retinal features when using FA, but it highlights well the microaneurysms, the dye leakage and staining. OCT angiography allows a clear vision of the small capillaries in the two vascular networks (superficial and deep)

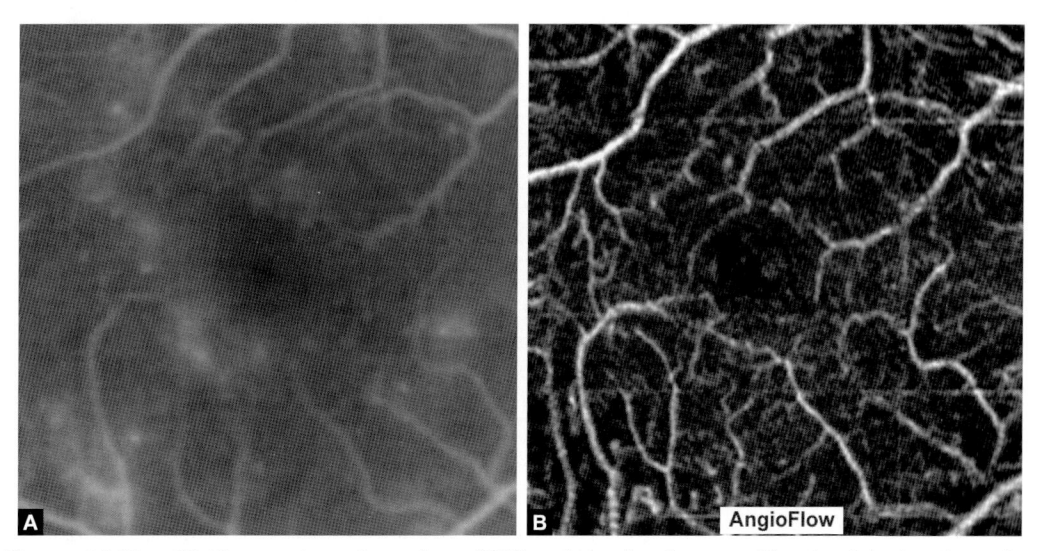

Figures 14.4A and B Fluorescein angiography and OCT angiography of a nonproliferative diabetic retinopathy. FA shows microaneurysms, dye leakage and staining. OCT angiography does not show all the microaneurysms but shows better the no flow areas

Noninvasive Method

It is possible to repeat OCT angiography frequently when needed, even in elderly people, in patients with cardiac diseases, and in pregnant women. This test is reassuring to both patients and their ophthalmologists as it is noninvasive.

Hyperfluorescence and Hypofluorescence in FA and Flow Signal in OCTA

In this section, we compare hyperfluorescence and hypofluorescence in images on FA and OCT angiography.

Hyperfluorescence Due to Fluorescein Angiography and Flow–vascular Signal in OCT Angiography

Window effect: The images on FA may present a window effect hyperfluorescence due to atrophy of the pigment screen that allows the observation of the deep and choroid layers. This effect may often interfere with the viewing of the retinal vasculature in front of it.

The OCT angiography selectively visualizes the layer to be studied without being influenced by the upper or lower layers. In case of the choroid, OCT angiography with normal pigment epithelium demonstrates the choriocapillaris with good resolution, while the medium and large-sized vessels appear to be black chords. In pigment epithelium atrophy, the choroid vessels are visualized in OCT angiography as white flowing signals, similar to the retinal vessels and with characteristics that are typical of the choroid.

Staining: FA shows hyperfluorescence due to staining that is usually rather uniform. OCT angiography is unable to visualize the vessel walls staining. However, it can indirectly demonstrate shading as seen by thickened walls and a reduction in flow.

Dye leakage: In the context of lesions responsible for dye leakage on FA, it is difficult to detect capillary networks, especially in cases of choroid neovascularization or of retinal, preretinal or prepapillary new vessels in ischemic retinopathies. The new vessels have a thin and highly permeable wall that tends to leak the dye in the earliest frames, resulting in blurring as the hyperfluorescence spreads out and masks the finer vessels. OCT cross-sections demonstrate fibrous or fibrovascular lesions as pseudostratified hyper-reflectant lesions or clearly branched lesions. OCT angiography at the level of the fibrous plaque often demonstrate neovascular branches within the fibrous lesions. The loop clusters of active new vessels are visualized clearly on OCT angiography both during the proliferating phase as well as during regression related to treatment.

Dye pooling: The lesions where dye accumulates on FA are not always visible on OCT angiography. These lesions, including microaneurysms, are visible on OCT angiography only when the flow inside the microaneurysm is fast enough to be detected. They are, otherwise, not evident on OCT-A even if they are present on FA. On the other hand, with OCT angiography it is possible to locate the aneurysm level precisely. These alterations can be observed mostly at the level of the deep vascular plexus. Failure to visualize these structures on OCT angiography may imply that the flow within is too fast (saturation limit), too slow (sensitivity limit) or absent as in thrombosed microaneurysms.

Nonperfused Areas on Fluorescein Angiography and OCT Angiography

Fluorescein Angiography: Hypofluorescence Due to Reduced or No Perfusion

Hypofluorescence caused by reduced perfusion or absent perfusion is a typical FA finding in ischemic areas. Ischemia is usually due to a reduction in the blood flow at the superficial vascular plexus level, while the deeper flow is frequently spared. This phenomenon decreases fluorescence in the ischemic areas on FA.

OCT Angiography: In Low Flow or no-flow Areas

In OCT Angiography, the ischemic area produces two typical alterations.

There is homogenization of the texture of the ischemic territory. In OCT angiography most of the ischemic areas (surface analysis, thickness 60-micron, and offset 6–15 micron) appear to have a low and rather uniform granular density, without evidence of flow.

Sometimes, important vessels disappear and only the large-sized vessels persist. As a result the smaller secondary and tertiary branches may not be seen.

The OCT angiography demonstrates vascular networks with obvious areas of no-flow that grossly correspond to the nonperfused areas on fluorescein angiography. The ischemic areas are zones where there are capillary dropouts, or capillaries are thinned out. These ischemic zones are more evident against a gray background. Often the capillaries inside the non-perfused areas appear as truncated, abrupt interruptions, arterio-venous shunts, or shunts with the deeper capillary layers of the deep vascular network (at the inner nuclear layer). These images appear sharper as there is no masking by dye leakage as in the intermediate and late frames of FA. The vascular network is therefore seen more sharply, and the arteriovenous shunts, the duplications and the vascular loops are seen more clearly. Above all, OCT angiography highlights details that cannot be seen with fluorescein angiography since there is no role for dye (**Figs 14.5A and B**).

Anomalous Vessels on Fluorescein Angiography

In case of ischemic exudative vascular disorders like diabetic retinopathy and venous occlusions, FA may show vessels that look truncated with hyperfluorescent staining on vascular walls and

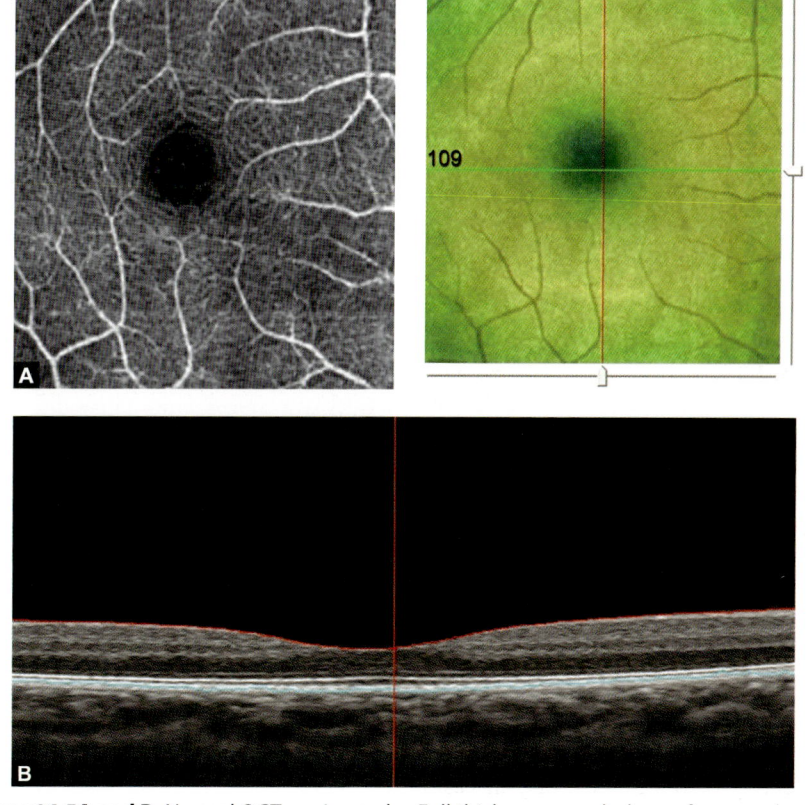

Figures 14.5A and B Normal OCT angiography. Full thickness morphology of a normal macula. The vascular aspects seen in this image correspond to the inner retinal network

late dye leakage. Some major vessels appear to be very thick because it is not possible to differentiate between hyperfluorescence due to wall staining and hyperfluorescence that reflects the dye inside the lumen.

Anomalous Vessels on OCT Angiography

Vascular branches of larger sizes may appear to be thick on fluorescein angiography because it is not possible to differentiate between hyperfluorescence caused by staining of the walls, and hyperfluorescence due to dye content.

In OCT angiography, these same vessels appear thinner than in FA, and generally show a dark para-axial sleeve-like streak. This dark sleeve-like shadow is the negative representation of the vessel wall that is hyperfluorescent on FA.

Special attention needs to be paid when assessing capillary dropout. It is likely that the apparently truncated vessels may have undergone a change in course, dipping deeper to the deep plexus to form compensatory shunts. The new course of the vessel could continue beyond the segmentation slice, thus giving the false impression of a truncated vessel. It is therefore necessary to shift the segmentation dynamically towards the outer retina to follow the course of the vessel and to establish the presence or absence of an interruption.

In occlusive disorders, it is possible that the deep vascular plexus may attempt to compensate the acute hypo perfusion of the superficial vascular plexus through large branches connecting the two plexuses.

At the level of the deep vascular plexus, there is texture rarefaction with larger residual vessels in a decidedly low-density texture. Frequently, there are vessel duplications, with loops of capillaries and vessel dilatations, which are more evident in the border region between the ischemic area and the normally perfused area.

The OCT angiography analysis of these vessels shows additional characteristics that are very important.

Presence of a black border around the vessel walls.

By reducing the thickness of the surface scan from 60 microns to 30 microns with the ILM profile, and by moving the offset towards the choroid at 15 micron steps, vessels are observed to take origin from the larger superficial vessels and extend down towards the outer retina. These vessels frequently appear to be thicker compared to the main retinal vessels. This perception is probably because their course is more parallel to the incident light while the larger vessels are perpendicular. Alternatively, this could be because of bifurcations without pericytes (flow regulation). These small vascular trunks link the superficial vascular plexus to the deep vascular plexus at level of the outer plexiform layer. The appearance of this plexus is thus heavily altered. The typical distribution here is replaced by a disorderly network of vessels whose sizes are irregularly altered, with densities that are not uniform and with evidence of no-flow areas.

Hypofluorescence Due to Masking

Retinal hemorrhages are seen as areas of slight masking but they are less evident than on fluorescein angiography where the hemorrhages conceal the posterior layers. Retinal edema may have a mild masking effect on fluorescein angiography, while on OCT angiography it results in blurred, thinned out capillaries that are less evident against the gray background. The OCT angiography images are similar but different from FA images.

The OCT angiography demonstrates the morphology of the vessels in a given layer without issues of dye pooling, staining, and leakage and without a window effect as seen on FA.

The sensitivity to masking of OCT angiography is different from that of the traditional FA. Indeed, the SSADA analyses the differences and lack of vascular signal **(Tables 14.1 and 14.2)**.

The Two Retinal Vascular Plexuses

In FA, the superficial and deep vascular plexuses are seen simultaneously and superimposed and overlaid on each other, making it impossible to selectively examine them. Fluorescein angiography highlights, almost exclusively, the superficial plexus and does not allow evaluation of the deep plexus. FA is a dynamic examination where the time-variable is closely linked to the definition of the lesions.

The OCT angiography is independent of the time factor in that it does not study the dynamics

Table 14.1 Some details are better seen with SSADA OCT angiography
• Superficial retinal capillaries are better seen with OCT angiography
• Deep retinal capillaries are seen only with OCT angiography
• Vertical anastomoses between plexuses are seen only with OCT angiography
• Peri-foveal arcades are seen better with OCT angiography
• The lack of leakage makes it possible to better visualize capillary anomalies, pre-retinal, sub-retinal and sub-choroid newly formed vessels (classic and occult)
• The lack of staining makes it possible to better see the anomalies of the vascular network
• Possibility to quantify CNV
• Possibility to quantify retinal vascularization

Abbreviations: SSADA, split-spectrum amplitude-decorrelation angiography; OCT, optical coherence tomography

Table 14.2 Some details not seen with SSADA OCT angiography
• Leakage, staining and pooling are not seen
• Exudates and microaneurysms are either not seen or are hard to see

Abbreviations: SSADA, split-spectrum amplitude-decorrelation angiography; OCT, optical conerence tomography

of the dye but detects blood flow inside the vessels. It highlights the superficial plexus very clearly and makes it possible to assess the deep plexus separately from the superficial plexus.

CNV and Preretinal New Vessels (Figs 14.6A and B)

In ischemic retinopathies, the neovascularization of the choroid, retina, and preretinal and prepapillary new vessels present a thin and highly permeable wall with early dye leakage in early FA frames. Their arborization branches cannot be seen due to masking by fluorescein leakage.

The OCT cross-section study shows fibrous and fibrovascular lesions as pseudostratified or having arborescent hyperreflectivity.

The OCT angiography performed at the level of the CNV neovascular membrane or of the fibrous plaque often highlights the small neovascular branches inside the arborization or within the fibrous lesions. The peripheral loops of the new vessels are clearly seen on OCT angiography both during natural progression as well as regression following treatment.

Other Noninvasive Angiography Techniques

Retinal function imaging (RFI): This system uses a strong light on the retina with stroboscopic flashes to highlight the erythrocytes in the capillaries. OCT with phase variance offers a very good view of the capillary layers.

Adaptive optics provides excellent images but the field is very limited and the capture time is long. Numerous adaptive optics images need to be collected in order to study a single area.

CONCLUSION

The OCT angiography with SSADA algorithm offers a three-dimensional view of the retina and highlights at least two micro vascular layers at the level of the ganglion cells and the inner nuclear layer. The capture time is very quick and the device exploits a postprocessing algorithm that reduces artefacts due to motion (Motion Correction Technology). OCT angiography provides the possibility of quantifying retinal vascularization and CNV.

AngioVue, at present, cannot completely replace fluorescein angiography.

Most ophthalmologists do not consider AngioVue as a simple angiography device, but as an improved version of OCT and include OCT angiography as a part of a complete OCT examination.

A limited compensation of the deficiencies of OCT angiography could be achieved by overlaying vascularization maps and thickness maps to demonstrate leaking capillaries.

However, the difference between fluorescein angiography and OCT angiography will not

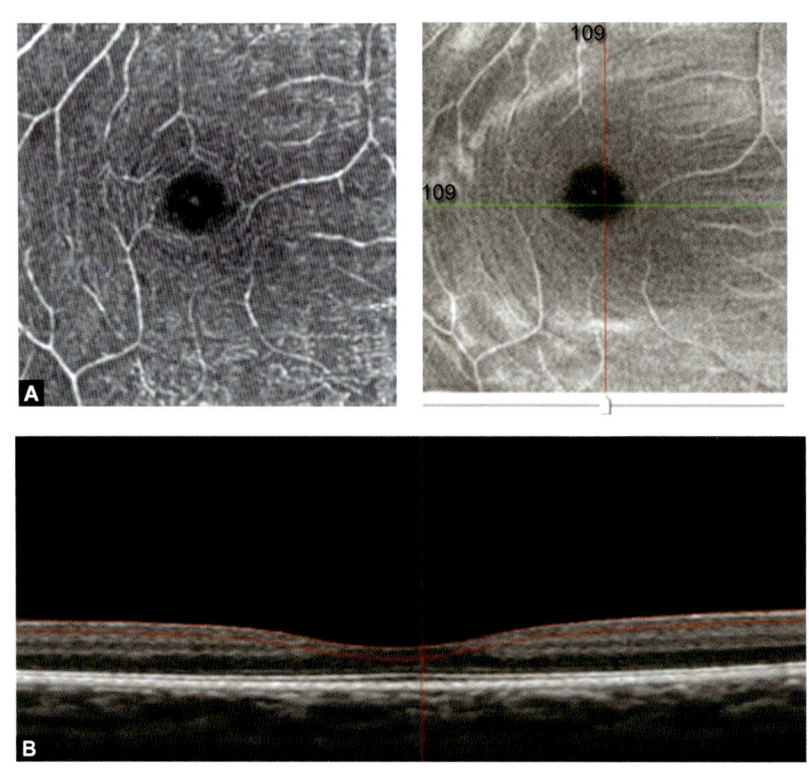

Figures 14.6A and B Normal OCT angiography. Morphology of the superficial plexus. Note how the segmentation is parallel to the retinal surface inner limiting membrane (ILM) with a thickness that is distant from the deep plexus, which therefore, is not seen. The main retinal vessels and the capillaries can be clearly seen immersed in a texture having medium reflectance

change as seen in routine hospital or office practice. FA is still sometimes necessary for the evaluation of retinal inflammation as in uveitis, choroiditis, many dubious retinopathies, and CSC. FA is still essential to settle difficult diagnosis and provide useful information in diabetic retinopathy and vein occlusion. The biggest advantage of OCT angiography is the possibility to quantify retinal vascularization and choroidal neovascularization (CNV).

BIBLIOGRAPHY

1. de Castro-Abeger AH, de Carlo TE, Duker JS, Baumal CR. Optical Coherence Tomography Angiography Compared to Fluorescein Angiography in Branch Retinal Artery Occlusion. Ophthalmic Surg Lasers Imaging Retina. 2015; 46(10):1052-4. doi: 10.3928/23258160-20151027-12.
2. Pauleikhoff D, Heimes B, Spital G, et al. OCT Angiography—Is this the Future for Macular Diagnosis? Klin Monbl Augenheilkd. 2015; 232(9):1069-76.

Index

Page numbers followed by *f* refer to figure

A

Age-related macular degeneration 48*f*, 61, 77, 87, 93*f*, 94
American Academy of Ophthalmology 28
Amplitude-decorrelation angiograms 2*f*
Angioid streaks 61
Antivascular endothelial growth factor 93
Arterial branch occlusions 39, 39*f*
Arterialization 50
Arteriolar branch occlusion 42
Avascular foveal zone 37

B

Branch retinal vein occlusion 36, 108*f*
Bruch's membrane 6, 50, 53*f*, 61, 108

C

Capillary density 45
Central retinal
  artery occlusion 40
  vein occlusion 33, 37, 38*f*
Central serous chorioretinopathy 61, 77, 89
  chronic 61, 70*f*, 72*f*, 73*f*
Central vein occlusions 33
Choriocapillaris 6
  segmentation 94*f*
Choroid 8
  capillary 8
Choroidal neovascularization 8, 10, 14*f*, 44, 45, 50, 53, 57, 61, 87, 89, 94, 95, 108*f*, 114
  types of 87
Choroiditis
  multiple 61
  scars of 74*f*
Cystoid macular edema 28, 30*f*

D

Deep plexus 25
Deep retinal capillaries 113
  plexus 8
Deep retinal plexus 6
Deep vascular plexus 20, 35
Degenerative myopia 61
  choroidal neovascularization of 62*f*
Diabetic retinopathy 28, 30*f*, 31*f*
  study 19
Dry age-related macular degeneration 9
Dyslipidemia 28

F

Fibrotic membrane 54, 54*f*
Fibrous scar 100
Fluorescein angiography 33, 36, 46, 48, 51, 52, 56*f*, 57, 57*f*, 61, 62*f*, 63*f*, 67*f*, 70*f*, 88, 103, 107, 108, 108*f*, 109*f*, 110, 111
Foveal avascular zone 8, 28

G

Ganglion cell complex 103
Glaucoma 103
Granular hyperfluorescences, multiple 89

H

Hemorrhages 38*f*, 91*f*
  multiple 88
  subretinal 14*f*
Hyperfluorescence 49, 110, 112

I

Indocyanine green angiography 3, 57, 57*f*-59*f*, 61, 63*f*, 70*f*, 77, 84*f*

Inner retinal blood flows, quantification of 10*f*
Intraretinal fluid 47
Ischemic maculopathy 30*f*, 31*f*

M

Macula 2*f*
Macular telangiectasia 90*f*
Medusa head 45
Multifocal choroiditis 61, 62, 74*f*-76*f*
Multimodal retinal imaging 90*f*, 91*f*
Myopia 52, 87
Myopic neovascular membrane 53*f*

N

Neovascular age-related macular degeneration 56
Neovascular membrane 17*f*, 52, 99
Nonproliferative diabetic retinopathy 109*f*

O

Optic nerve 103
  head 103
Optical coherence tomography (OCT) 1, 2, 2*f*, 6, 10, 14, 16, 28, 29*f*, 61, 88, 103, 107, 113
  angiography 1, 6, 7*f*, 10, 16, 22, 24, 28, 31*f*, 33, 34, 46, 47*f*, 48*f*, 49, 49*f*, 50-52, 52*f*, 53, 53*f*, 56, 58, 63*f*-65*f*, 69*f*, 72*f*, 93, 93*f*, 98, 103, 104*f*, 107, 109, 109*f*, 110, 112
  limitations of 3
  principles of 1
  noninvasive 44

P

Pachychoroid diseases 77
Paracentral acute middle maculopathy 40

Peripapillary branch retinal artery occlusion 41*f*
Pigment epithelial detachment 77*f*
Pigment epithelium 50
Plexiform layer 24
Polypoidal choroidal vasculopathy 77, 91*f*
Polypoidal saccular dilatations 84*f*
Proliferative diabetic retinopathy 11*f*
Pseudoxanthoma elasticum 61

Q

Quantify retinal vascularization 113

R

Retinal angiomatous proliferations 91*f*
Retinal artery occlusion 40, 41
Retinal edema 33, 37
Retinal function imaging 113
Retinal ischemia 37, 38, 38*f*
Retinal neovascularization 10, 11
  detection of 10
Retinal nerve fiber layer 103
Retinal pigment epithelium 3, 23, 57, 77, 94
Retinal vascular networks 24

S

Scanning laser ophthalmoscopy 77
Spectral domain optical coherence tomography 57, 94
Split-spectrum amplitude decorrelation angiography 1, 6, 16, 24, 28, 34, 44, 103, 113
Subretinal fibrosis 93, 93*f*, 94*f*, 96*f*
Subretinal pigment epithelium 11
Superficial layer 51
Superficial plexus 25
Superficial retinal capillaries 113
  plexus 8
Superficial retinal plexus 6
Superficial vascular plexus 18, 18*f*, 24, 34

V

Vascular density map 18, 20
Vascular fibrosis 95
Venous branch occlusion 33
Vitreous 6

W

White line artifacts 22

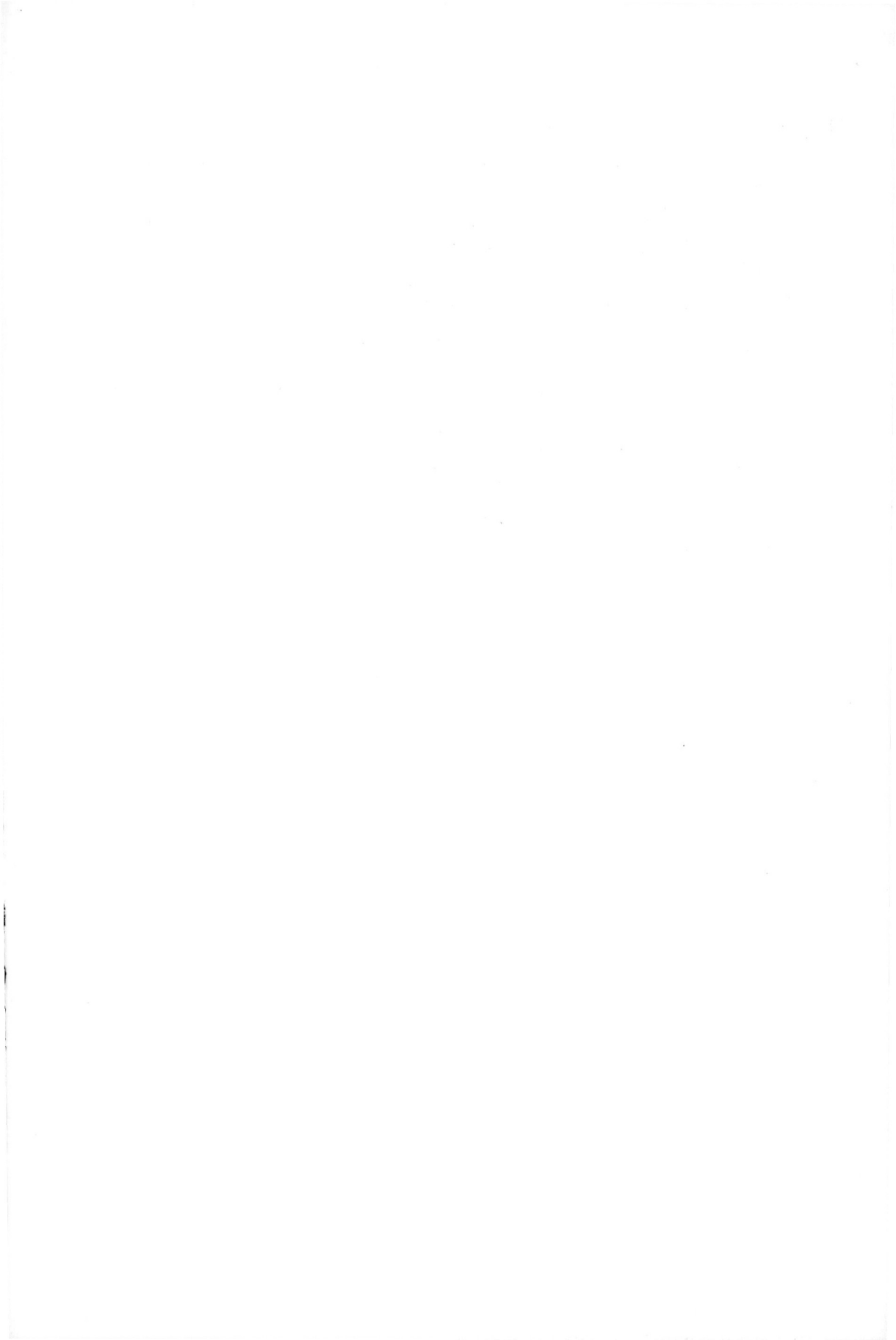